The Resonant Connection
Integrating Qi Coil Technology with Chiropractic Care

Dr. Bill Ormston, D.V,M., AVCA Certified Animal Chiropractor

The Resonant Connection: Integrating Qi Coil Technology with Chiropractic Care

Dr. Bill Ormston, D.V,M., AVCA Certified Animal Chiropractor

Copyright 2024. Wm. L. Ormston, DVM. Meridian, Texas

All rights reserved. No part of this booklet may be reproduced or transmitted in any form or by any means, electronic or mechanical, including photocopy, recording or any other information technology without the prior permission in writing from the author.

Introduction
- Questioning Conventional Veterinary Practices
- Historical and Scientific Context of Disease and Prevention
- Personal Catalyst for Exploring Alternatives
- Rediscovering Foundational Natural Principles

Part I: The Foundation of Healing Frequencies

Chapter 1: The History of Energy and Frequency Medicine
- The origins of magnetic healing and D.D. Palmer's early experiments.
- The evolution from static magnetism to pulsed electromagnetic fields (PEMF).
- Rife frequencies, Tesla's resonance theories, and the modern quantum perspective.
- The emergence of portable frequency devices—where Qi Coil fits in.

Chapter 2: Chiropractic and Energy: Parallel Philosophies
- The 33 Principles and the flow of Universal Intelligence.
- Nerve interference and subluxation as vibrational distortion.
- Chiropractic's innate intelligence and frequency coherence.
- Why vibration, tone, and resonance are central to both chiropractic and energy medicine.

Chapter 3: The Science of Resonance and Cellular Communication
- Bioelectric fields and piezoelectricity in the body.
- Frequency-specific tissue response: mitochondria, nerves, and fascia.
- Brainwave entrainment and coherence in humans and animals.
- Evidence base for PEMF and frequency therapy: key studies and mechanisms.

Part II: The Qi Coil System Explained

Chapter 4: The Qi Coil Design and Technology
- Structure and engineering: toroidal field design and Tesla coil principles.
- Differences between Qi Coil, Bemer, Magna Wave, and Assisi Loop.
- Scalar energy, harmonic resonance, and the concept of "no-contact" therapy.
- Frequency generation: app-controlled precision and waveform modulation.

Chapter 5: Frequency Sets and Healing Applications
- Overview of frequency categories: detox, immune, pain, regeneration, emotional balance.
- Understanding Rife-derived sets and harmonic stacking.
- How the Qi Coil app organizes and delivers therapeutic programs.
- Case examples of physical and behavioral transformation.

Chapter 6: Clinical Evidence, Case Studies, and the Future of Frequency-Based Chiropractic
    Scientific Foundations and Evidence.
    Veterinary Applications and Case Studies.
    Integration, Education, and Future Directions.

Part III: Integration with Chiropractic Practice

Chapter 7: The Philosophy of Resonance: Integrating Mind, Matter, and Motion
    Resonance as Chiropractic's Philosophical Core.
    Mind–Body–Field Integration.
    Ethics and the Art of Practice.
    From Individual Coherence to Ecological Harmony:

Chapter 8, Applied Resonance: Practice, Community, and Continuity
    Translating Resonance Theory into Daily Practice:
    Integration Across Species and Professions:
    Ethics, Economics, and Evidence:
    Expanding Circles of Coherence:

Chapter 9, Energy-Field Coherence and Chiropractic Philosophy
    The Body as a Resonant Network.
    Integration of Mechanics and Electromagnetics.
    Coherence Across Practitioners, Patients, and Environments.
    Reframing chiropractic care as "neuromagnetic realignment."

Chapter 10: The Resonant Doctor — Living the Chiropractic Way of Being
    Embodying the Frequency
    The Discipline of Daily Coherence
    Listening, Service, and Ethical Resonance
    Mastery, Mentorship, and Legacy

Chapter 11: The Living Field — Humanity, Animals, and the Future of Conscious Care
    Healing as a Shared Field
    From Mechanistic Thinking to Resonant Ecology
    Reciprocity, Ethics, and Technology
    Toward Planetary and Photonic Consciousness

Part IV: Building the Integrative Future

Chapter 12: The Continuum of Light Practice, Presence, and the Infinite Field
- The Practitioner as Living Laboratory
- Communities of Resonance and Ethical Governance
- Art, Stillness, and Compassion as Scientific Forces
- The Infinite Feedback Loop — Evolution as Adjustment

Chapter 13: Applied Resonance – Tools, Protocols, and Integration Models.
- The Five-Step Resonant Integration Model
- Rhythmic Scheduling and Field Application
- Multimodal Resonance Therapies and Layered Protocols
- Client Education, Compliance, and Outcome Tracking

Chapter 14 Living in Coherence — The Practitioner as the Field
- The Doctor as Environment
- Practitioner Self-Care and Energy Hygiene
- Developing Intuitive Resonance
- Translating and Teaching Coherence

Appendices

Appendix A: Glossary of Vibrational Medicine Terms.
Appendix B: Frequency Reference Charts (common sets and targets).
Appendix C: Owner's Observation Log
Appendix D: QiCoil Canine Protocols Short
Appendix E: QiCoil Canine Protocols Long
Appendix E: QiCoil Feline Protocols Short
Appendix F: QiCoil Equine Protocols Short
Appendix G: QiCoil Equine Protocols Long
Appendix H: A to Z QiCoil Animal Protocols
Appendix I: Comparative Cost and Setup Guide (Qi Coil vs. other PEMF).

Introduction

The introduction establishes Dr. O's transformation from a traditionally trained veterinarian into a holistic practitioner guided by inquiry rather than convention. By juxtaposing unquestioned medical norms with the demand for deeper understanding, he invites readers to rethink what "science-based care" truly means. His personal story—anchored in both professional rigor and parental urgency—illustrates how disillusionment can evolve into enlightenment. Through critical reflection on medicine's historical biases and the enduring relevance of natural laws, Dr. O sets the stage for why devices like the Qi Coil represent not pseudoscience, but a return to foundational truths about energy, resonance, and life itself.

PART I: The Foundation of Healing Frequencies

Chapter 1: The History of Energy and Frequency Medicine

This chapter opens by tracing the roots of energy-based healing from ancient magnetism to D.D. Palmer's early experiments with magnetic healing in the late 1800s. It follows the evolution of therapeutic magnetism through Tesla's discoveries of alternating current and resonant fields, the refinement of electromagnetic therapy in the 20th century, and the rise of Rife frequencies and PEMF technology. The chapter concludes by showing how modern innovations like the Qi Coil system build upon this legacy—transforming once-static magnetic therapies into dynamic, frequency-controlled systems that support biological healing.

Chapter 2: Chiropractic and Energy—Parallel Philosophies

Chiropractic and energetic medicine share a foundational belief: life is governed by tone, vibration, and flow. This chapter explores the parallels between the chiropractic concept of Innate Intelligence and the vibrational theories of resonance and coherence. It discusses how subluxation represents a disruption in the body's energetic flow, and how adjustment—like frequency therapy—restores order and communication. Through the lens of the 33 Principles, readers see how both chiropractic and frequency healing ultimately seek to reconnect the organism with its vital source.

Chapter 3: The Science of Resonance and Cellular Communication

Modern biology confirms what early chiropractors intuited: cells communicate through subtle electrical and magnetic signals. This chapter examines the science of bioelectricity, piezoelectric properties of bone and fascia, and the role of electromagnetic signaling in tissue repair. It explores how specific frequencies influence ion channels, mitochondrial activity, and neural pathways. Supported by studies in PEMF, EEG coherence, and cellular resonance, it provides the physiological framework that explains why frequency-based technologies like Qi Coil complement manual chiropractic adjustments.

PART II: The Qi Coil System Explained

Chapter 4: The Qi Coil Design and Technology

Readers are introduced to the engineering behind the Qi Coil. The toroidal coil structure generates a scalar magnetic field that penetrates tissue without direct contact. This chapter compares the Qi Coil to other PEMF devices such as Bemer, Magna Wave, and Assisi Loop, highlighting differences in waveform design, frequency modulation, and portability. It explains the Tesla-inspired physics behind its operation and how the mobile app controls precise frequency output, making this technology accessible for both clinical and home use.

Chapter 5: Frequency Sets and Healing Applications

Each frequency carries a unique biological signature. This chapter explores how the Qi Coil organizes frequencies into targeted programs—for pain relief, immune enhancement, cellular regeneration, and emotional balance. It outlines the concept of harmonic stacking and frequency layering to amplify outcomes. Clinical and anecdotal examples illustrate improved mobility, calmer behavior, and faster recovery in both human and animal patients when specific frequency protocols are combined with chiropractic care.

Chapter 6: Clinical Evidence, Case Studies, and the Future of Frequency-Based Adjusting.

This chapter charts the evolution of animal chiropractic from philosophical origins to a scientifically grounded discipline. It compiles research demonstrating how pulsed electromagnetic fields (PEMF) and chiropractic adjustments synergistically enhance healing, neurological function, and stress regulation across species. Through equine, canine, and bovine case studies, the chapter shows measurable outcomes in mobility, recovery, and productivity supported by objective markers like HRV, EMG symmetry, and cortisol reduction. Methodological rigor and ethical responsibility are positioned as the foundation for future research. The chapter concludes by envisioning a profession that unites technological precision with practitioner coherence—where resonance-based care not only advances veterinary medicine but also contributes to broader goals of animal welfare, sustainability, and regenerative agriculture.

PART III: Integration with Chiropractic Practice

Chapter 7, The Philosophy of Resonance: Integrating Mind, Matter, and Motion

This chapter brings chiropractic full circle; back to its vibrational roots while aligning it with modern science. It interprets classic principles such as the Law of Tone and Innate Intelligence through measurable concepts like coherence, heart-rate variability, and electromagnetic entrainment. By linking emotion, physiology, and field resonance, the chapter portrays chiropractic touch and frequency-based therapies as complementary waveforms restoring harmony in living systems. Ethical practice, emotional awareness, and intuitive presence remain central, ensuring that technology amplifies rather than replaces the human element. Expanding the vision further, resonance is shown to operate from cellular to ecological scales, positioning the chiropractor as both healer and steward of coherence across animals, herds, and the living planet. Ultimately, the chapter envisions a unified paradigm where science, philosophy, and compassion converge—keeping life, quite literally, in tune.

Chapter 8, Applied Resonance: Practice, Community, and Continuity.

The reader learns how chiropractic transforms the science of resonance into a living philosophy of care. It outlines how coherent principles shape everything from clinic design and daily rhythm to multispecies protocols and community outreach. By blending chiropractic adjustments with frequency-based therapies in ethically grounded, evidence-supported practice, the resonant chiropractor becomes both healer and educator. The chapter emphasizes collaboration with veterinarians, honest communication with clients, and self-maintenance to preserve clinical sensitivity. Beyond individual outcomes, it reveals resonance as a unifying force linking practitioner well-being, client trust, herd stability, and ecological renewal. Ultimately, applied resonance is portrayed as chiropractic's fullest expression—philosophy in action, harmonizing the self, the clinic, the community, and the planet.

Chapter 9, Energy-Field Coherence and Chiropractic Philosophy.

This chapter unites chiropractic's vitalistic origins with contemporary biophysics and veterinary science. It presents the body as a resonant network in which mechanical motion, electromagnetic flow, and consciousness operate as one system. Chiropractic adjustments and frequency-based therapies re-tune this network, restoring coherence from cell to herd to ecosystem. Scientific evidence—from HRV synchronization to biophoton emission and PEMF outcomes—supports the principle that healing is the reorganization of energy, not the suppression of symptoms. The chapter concludes that the future of chiropractic lies in mastering both the physics of resonance and the ethics of coherence, empowering practitioners to serve as custodians of alignment for animals, humans, and the living planet itself.

Chapter 10: The Resonant Doctor — Living the Chiropractic Way of Being

Chapter 10 reframes chiropractic not as a profession but as a state of being. The resonant doctor integrates science, service, and spirit through coherence—living as both practitioner and instrument. Daily discipline, empathic listening, ethical integrity, and collaborative mentorship weave together to form a lifestyle of alignment. In this model, every breath, adjustment, and act of service becomes a broadcast of harmony that ripples from individual to community to world. To "live the chiropractic way of being" is to embody the adjustment itself—a steady, compassionate vibration within the greater field of life.

Chapter 11: The Living Field — Humanity, Animals, and the Future of Conscious Care

Chapter 11 envisions a world where chiropractic care expands into planetary stewardship. It portrays a future in which the boundaries between human, animal, and environment dissolve into one luminous network of coherence. Through conscious technology, ethical intention, and interspecies empathy, the resonant doctor participates in Earth's own healing. Light, frequency, and compassion converge into a single science of connection. In this vision, every adjustment—whether of spine, circuit, or society—becomes a prayer of alignment, restoring rhythm to the living field that sustains all life.

PART IV: Building the Integrative Future

Chapter 12: The Continuum of Light - Practice, Presence, and the Infinite Field

Chapter 12 closes the book while opening the field. It calls the reader to live research—to treat every breath, patient, and encounter as data in the grand experiment of coherence. The resonant doctor becomes a living instrument, attuned to both measurable and mystical realities. Through community, artistry, silence, and compassionate awareness, practice transcends profession and becomes prayer. In this perpetual feedback loop of learning and evolution, chiropractic emerges as a way of being that harmonizes body, mind, and planet. Healing, at its highest octave, is simply love in resonance.

Chapter 13: Applied Resonance – Tools, Protocols, and Integration Models

Chapter 13 bridges philosophy and practice, turning the abstract beauty of resonance into tangible systems for everyday use. Through the Five-Step Resonant Integration Model, rhythmic scheduling, multimodal therapies, and client-centered education, applied resonance becomes both science and ceremony. Every tool—from Qi Coil to PEMF—is integrated within a coherent framework that honors chiropractic principles while embracing modern technology. The result is a practice culture where frequency, intention, and rhythm unite—making each adjustment not only a correction but a contribution to global coherence.

Chapter 14 Living in Coherence — The Practitioner as the Field

Chapter 14 concludes the journey from principle to embodiment. It calls the practitioner to become the very field through which healing flows—a coherent presence whose physiology, intention, and awareness radiate order into every environment. Through disciplined self-care, intuitive development, clear teaching, and vibrational precision, the chiropractor transforms from technician to transmitter. Living in coherence means practicing what chiropractic has always proclaimed: that life heals when interference—

whether spinal, emotional, or energetic—is removed. The coherent doctor does not merely adjust the spine; they tune the symphony of life itself.

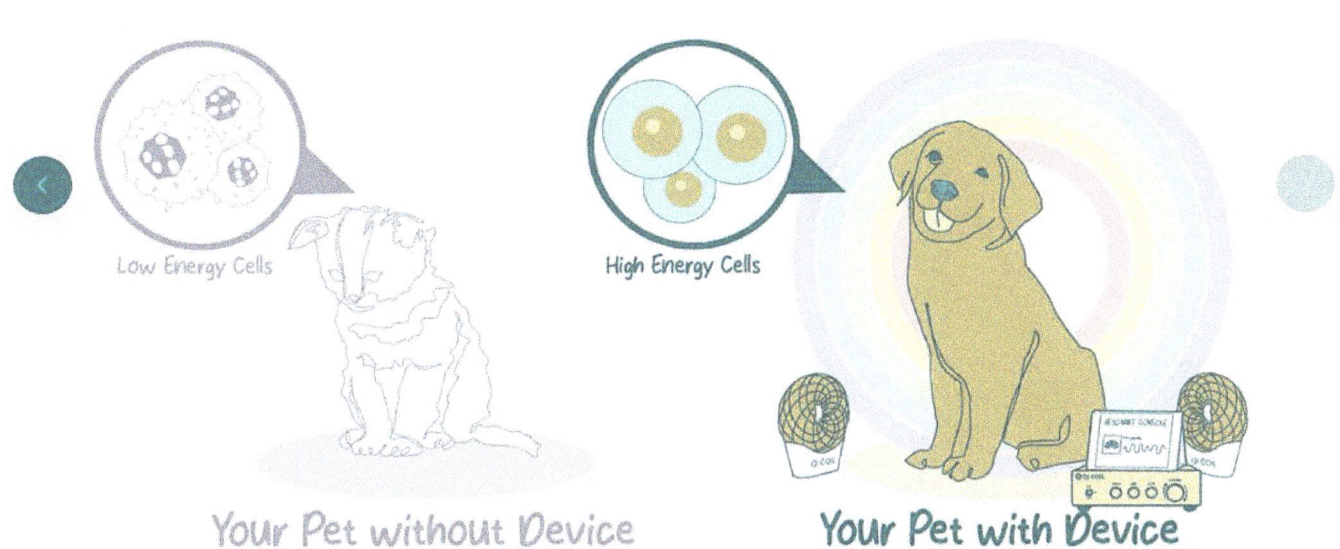

"Hello, my name is Dr. O. I have been a veterinarian for over 36 years. You need to purchase a Qi-Coil to ensure your pet's maximum health and well-being."

"What?", you are asking. If I had told you to buy some medications or get a series of vaccinations for your pet, we would be done already. You would be on the way to the cashier confident in the fact that your veterinarian had done what was necessary to keep your pet healthy for as long as possible. But if I introduce something new that you haven't heard of before, you start to ask questions. Questions that should be asked of all medical professionals about any products that they are recommending.

Why? Should I give my dog heartworm pills? The first reported case of heartworms in the United States was in 1847. The first preventative was marketed in 1977, and the Incidence of heartworm disease has continued to rise not only in previously known hot spots but also in unexpected locations with previously low heartworm rates, according to the 2022 Heartworm Incidence Map from the American Heartworm Society (AHS). Heartworms don't infect healthy dogs, just dogs full of chronic inflammation.

Why? Should I get those routine vaccinations every year. Dog vaccines are protective for some diseases, like parvovirus, but overvaccination can definitely lead to problems with chronic diseases. Because veterinarians are taught in school that the science says vaccinate often to protect everyone.

Why? When I started looking at alternative methods to treat my own son who had developed epilepsy 9 hours after his third MMR shot, was I not informed that seizures could be a side effect of the vaccination. As I looked into things that other people had good results using on their relatives with seizures, I was constantly told that the science wasn't good, those products are old fashioned and if you don't treat your son the way we say, we might just take him away.

I had forgotten to ask questions as I was studying to get my Doctor of Veterinary Medicine, but I started asking more questions as I searched for answers to help my family. Why weren't some of these very effective treatment protocols used anymore? Why did we need to learn many of the laws of physics and chemistry, and then learn pharmacology where we were told the laws of nature don't really matter.

As I found the answers to some of these questions, I went through the five stages of grief: denial, anger, bargaining, depression, and acceptance. I also found the reason that you need to purchase a Qi-Coil to ensure your pet's maximum health and well-being.

At first, I was in denial due to the fact that I had just spent eight years in school studying the newest and best procedures and medications in order to pass the veterinary board exam and begin to practice veterinary medicine. If these other modalities existed and did work as people claimed, why weren't they taught in veterinary school. The other stages are intermingled as I researched these treatment methods and began to understand more about the whys. A short history lesson may be in order.

Verywell Mind is a web site hosted by board-certified physicians that verify the medical accuracy of the articles on their site and they state that alternative therapies refer to any medical treatments that are not traditional medicine techniques. Alternative therapies could either be used alongside conventional medicine or instead of it. The term is often used interchangeably with "complementary medicine." In medical spaces, the practice is referred to as Complementary and Alternative Medicine (CAM).[1] The National Institutes of Health (NIH) does make a distinction between complementary and alternative medicine. According to them, when it's used alongside traditional medicine, it's complementary, but if it's used in place of conventional medicine, then it's considered alternative.[2] However, most people are likely to use these therapies alongside traditional medicine. When a licensed healthcare provider uses both alternative therapies and conventional medicine, then it's called integrative medicine.[3] A doctor or healthcare provider who uses integrative medicine uses all therapeutic methods to ensure their patients are healthy. Sometimes treatments may go from traditional to alternative or vice versa. When I was in veterinary school, glucosamine was considered alternative therapy and is now considered mainstream. Leeches were once a mainstay of medicine and fell out of favor but are making a comeback!![4] Whoa….

In the early 1900's there were 155 medical schools, 28 veterinary schools, 14 chiropractic schools and a few osteopathic schools. Two gentlemen (Rockefeller and Carnegie) were having difficulty introducing some of their new petrochemical biproducts into the medical realm. They decided if there was some standardization of medical education it would be easier to make changes. They funded the "Flexner Report". From January 1909, through April, 1910, Abraham Flexner traveled throughout the United States and Canada on a trip that revolutionized North American medical education. He visited every one of the existing 155 medical schools and, by the end of 1910, had published his report detailing the resources and practices of all these schools. Startlingly, he also recommended closing

---

[1] https://verywellmind.com/alternative-therapies-types-and-uses-5207962
[2] National Center for Complementary and Integrative Health. Complementary, alternative, or integrative health: what's in a name?.
[3] GETTING STARTED. What Are Alternative Therapies? Toketemu Ohwovoriole, November 08, 2021
[4] Younis Munshi, Irfat Ara, Huma Rafique and Zahoor Ahmad, 2008. Leeching in the History-A Review. Pakistan Journal of Biological Sciences, 11: 1650-1653.

120 of them. The report, commissioned by the Carnegie Foundation for the Advancement of Teaching, begins by projecting needs for well-educated physicians and then articulates the educational resources and standards necessary before proceeding to detail the specifics of each school.[5] Abraham's brother, Simon Flexner, was the head of the Rockefeller Institute for Medical Research.

Flexner divided the schools into three categories depending on the standards outlined in the first part of the report. In the first were those already meeting or about to meet all the standards. In the second were "almost rans", those able to meet the standards with reasonable and obtainable improvement. The remaining schools were lumped into the third and final category as essentially hopeless, with no reasonable expectation of ever meeting the standards. Subsequently, large numbers of schools were closed (although not 120) and the ones that remained increasingly adopted what has come to be known as the "Flexner Curriculum", essentially still in use today. While identified as the "Flexner" curriculum, Flexner simply describes, with appropriate citations, curricula originating in Berlin and Vienna (including a paper by a certain Theodore Billroth) which had already been summarized by the American Medical Association and the Association of American Medical Colleges. This curriculum was already standard in more than a dozen schools at the time, most famously Johns Hopkins. The New York School of Homeopathic Medicine failed, got a grant from the Carnegie Foundation, changed their name, added pharmacology and became the New York School of Medicine. They went from being the biggest educator of homeopathic medicine to a premiere pharmacology and research facility. Only two veterinary schools remained open.

The American Medical Association was formed in the early 1800's by physicians that chose to use drugs instead of herbs and more natural means. The Journal of the American Medical Association editor was also the head of the AMA during these early yrs.; Simmons headed the organizations from 1900-1924 and Fishbein from 1924-1949. George "Doc" Simmons was never a doctor, although he spent years in medical practice - he obtained a diploma by mail from Rush Medical College, a diploma mill. Fishbein did complete studies at a medical school, although he never completed his internship, never received a diploma, and never practiced medicine a day in his life. They both derisively labeled as "quacks" any alternative practitioner and used the full weight of the Journal to expose the practitioner as a fraud and get their work stopped.[6]

---

[5] How Abraham Flexner is Failing Surgery. September 22, 2017 by Association for Academic Surgery Webmaster
[6] A Brief and Sordid History of the American Medical Association and Modern Medicine. Dr. Michael Wayne. October 20, 2916

What Simmons and Fishbein had in common, besides a complete dictatorial control of the AMA and a hatred for all types of alternative modalities, was a desire to use their position to fatten their wallets through extortion. They had a deal with pharmaceutical companies, whereby they would give the AMA Seal of Approval on various drugs, if the drug companies made a substantial donation to the AMA; a portion of the donation went into the pockets of Simmons and then, after Simmons was forced to retire from the AMA, Fishbein. Since the AMA had no labs, no testing equipment, or any research staff, it was by the whim and decree of these two men what drugs got the Seal of Approval. Another ruse they had was to buy up huge sums of stock on drugs that they were about to give the Seal of Approval to. Once the approval was released, the stock price would go through the roof, and Simmons and Fishbein would reap the rewards. Simmons was forced to retire in 1924; Fishbein kept his stranglehold on the AMA until 1949, when he was kicked out.[7]

Morris Fishbein, M.D. is the most important non-chiropractor to influence the chiropractic profession. From his post as editor and secretary of the American Medical Association, his anti-chiropractic writings, speeches and political activities had a profound effect on the profession's development. Because he was not only the foremost medical politician of the time, but also perceived as a multi-faceted author on public health issues, his credibility was high across large sections of the population and in most social institutions. His tactics and stature undoubtedly helped keep the profession limited to caring for a small percentage of the population. Because of him, chiropractors devised survival strategies that continue to influence the profession even today.[8]

But the damage was done, and promising natural and holistic therapies were left in their wake. Instead, the public got Health, Incorporated, and were led to believe that only a doctor who practiced modern medicine knew what was best. We were told to follow the scientific validity of the AMA. Even during some huge viral outbreaks, we were told to follow the science by an organization whose biggest supporter until the 1950's was the tobacco industry. Much science was scoffed and tossed away as not valid, unless it was sold to the AMA.

In this same era Albert Einstein believed that the body was more than the sum of its parts and that electricity and magnetism is the basis of life. Energetic concepts of medicine have been described in all traditional medical philosophies throughout the world. In traditional Chinese medicine the primal energy is known as Qi, Chi, or Ki (pronounced chee). In homeopathy, it is known as the Vital Force. Energetic force creates order in living

---

[7] A Brief and Sordid History of the American Medical Association and Modern Medicine. Dr. Michael Wayne. October 20, 2916

[8] Donahue JH. Morris Fishbein, M.D.: the "medical Mussolini" and chiropractic. Chiropr Hist. 1996 Jun;16(1):39-49. PMID: 11619004.

systems and constantly rebuilds and renews cellular components. When the energetic force leaves the body at death, the physical body slowly decays and becomes a disorganized collection of chemicals. Energetic force is unique, distinguishing living from non-living systems and people from machines. Immunosuppression is a disorder at the electromagnetic and physical levels that manifest itself in the body in the form of symptoms. If the vital force of living is suppressed or lacking, there are no drugs or antibiotics that can cure the body. This unseen connection between spiritual and physical bodies must be understood and addressed if we are to understand health and illness.

Bioenergy conducts the process of healing and growth from birth to death. It can be controlled by the mind and communication between individuals. Because it flows in the direction from highest concentration to lowest, it can establish order from disorder, thus promoting healing. Every living being radiates energy, which is called the photon emission of living cells and is commonly called the aura. In a healthy cell, positive and negative cells are in balance. The cell membrane has a negative charge, the cytoplasm is neutral, and the nucleus is positively charged. Research has proven that bone growth and white blood cell activity can be affected by electricity. Increased activity and growth occur near a negative electrode and decreased activity and growth at the positive electrode. The chief aim of all healing methods should be directed towards the preservation, restoration and regeneration of the electrical potential. It is within the electrical potential of an organism that the key to curing and healing is found.

All of the varying alternative methods work on different energy levels. Some work on the physical level and cause responses on the same level. These methods are easier to prove scientifically. Homeopathic remedies are "vibrational medicines." If the remedy's frequency matches the patient's illness state, a resonant transfer of energy allows the patient's bioenergetic system to assimilate the needed energy, eliminate dissonant frequencies, and move to a new equilibrium of health. The etheric body holds the memories and experiences throughout all your animal's lifetime. Initially, it is meant to protect their physical body and is full of love and light along with a beautiful blueprint for their lifetime. Homeopathic remedies work on the etheric double. Flower essences work on the etheric and emotional range. Healing that takes place on energy levels filters down to the physical body. A cure is not complete until all levels are cleared. This explains why some dogs are triggered by things like a person in a cap or thunderstorms. This relates to an imbalance in the nervous system that requires deep healing, not just a temporary band-aid.

I started looking at alternative therapies when I realized that traditional medicine and medications were not really helping my epileptic son with his seizures. I bought numerous books on homeopathic medicine, herbal medicine, and many others. Each and every modality has some science or centuries old reasons for why they work. Let's take a brief look at some of the more common ones in use today. We use many of them in our practice, however modalities are only used after three chiropractic adjustments. Once I truly understood the benefits of chiropractic care and how and why the adjustment works, our holistic approach to health care started to make sense to me. When we look at a safety pin that is closed and think of the top as the brain or control center and one side of the pin as nerves going down and the other side of the pin as nerves coming into the brain, the closed pin works. Open the pin and the circuit is not complete. There are many modalities that will help the animal feel better or help mask the gap in the open safety pin, but only a very precise movement will close the safety pin completing the circuit. Only after removing the nervous system interferences do we decide to add additional therapies to the treatment plan of any animal. The information in this chapter is presented to help you understand how the different methods of therapies are designed to work with and on your dog. Each and every treatment modality has what is called a mechanism of action. In medical terminology, the term mechanism of action (MOA) refers to the specific biochemical interaction through which a product or substance produces its healing effect. A mechanism of action usually includes mention of the specific molecular targets to which the product binds, such as an enzyme or receptor. Receptor sites have specific affinities for treatment modalities based on the chemical structure of the product, as well as the specific action that occurs there. In contrast, a mode of action (MoA) describes functional or anatomical changes, at the cellular level, resulting from the exposure of a living organism to a substance. In alternative medicines the MOA are usually milder than with traditional drugs, however they all still work because of their MOA or the goal behind how they work. Chiropractic's MoA is to remove interference from the nervous system to allow the body to work at optimal levels.

The physical body that can be seen and touched has an energy twin called the etheric double. This is the first of the energy bodies or aura layers. Whatever the health state of the first aura is reflected in the animal's physical body. The second aura or energy level is the emotional body. The emotional being must be free of dis-ease for the physical body to be cured. Emotional pain leads to physical ailments. Effects of emotional abuse may last long after the abuse is removed. The mental body is the third aura. Many aberrant animal behaviors come from misguided thought processes. Remember that dogs and cats don't focus well on close up objects. They may have difficulty visually differentiating new people from the ones that abused them or caused them pain. Dis-ease may move from the physical body to the other energy levels or begin in the emotional or spiritual levels and filter down to the physical body. A dis-ease that is only in the physical body is easier to clear than one that has affected the spiritual and emotional levels. Pets are spiritual and have a oneness with the universe. If this oneness is disrupted, animals can and do grieve themselves to death.

The first alternative therapy that I looked into was Homeopathy. I bought numerous books in an attempt to find the correct homeopathic remedy to help my son with his seizures. Every one of the books that I bought explained that seizures were a serious issue and recommended that l contact a homeopath in my area. There were none and so I ended up with a degree in Veterinary Homeopathy from the British Institute of Homeopathic medicine. It turns out that the largest and most prestigious school of homeopathic medicine in the US had fallen victim to the Flexner report. "The Homeopathic Medical College of the State of New York in New York City." became "New York Medical College" in 1935 after the publication of the report.[9] Homeopathy is based on the law of similars which is often summarized by the Latin phrase, "similia similibus curantur," usually translated as "like shall cure like." Samuel Hahnemann devised the first so-called "provings," experimental tests of remedies on healthy individuals to document the homeopathic effect in 1796. Hippocrates (around 400BC) also said, "By similar things a disease is produced and through the application of the like is cured". I have used many homeopathic remedies both personally and to treat animals with fantastic results. It is postulated that homeopathic remedies contain an energy essence of the plant or other substance from which they are prepared. The energy essence of the homeopathic remedy carries a type of subtle-energy signature of a particular frequency.[10] The biggest issue with homeopathic is the large number of remedies that are available. There are currently over 8,000 remedies that have been proven available. The practicality of having the correct one of these on hand for every condition is unreasonable. The major side effect of not having the correct remedy was that I wasted the patients time in healing and didn't help them in their attempt to return to health.

The impracticality of having the correct remedy on hand is what piqued my interest to cold laser therapy when one of my mentors, Dr. Rick Kauffman explained that the Erchonia cold laser and now the AVANT cold laser pulse at the frequency that you select. You may select any frequency that you wish and almost all homeopathic remedies have a known Rife frequency. I didn't know who Rife was at the time, but knew that changing vibration was important. This was an awesome improvement from the simple homeopathic remedies that I was using for a couple of reasons. The first improvement was that I could program up to four or eight frequencies at one time that were rotated over a three-minute treatment

_____

[9] https://www.nymc.edu/about/history/
[10] Vibrational Medicine. Richard Gerber, MD. 2001

protocol and the treatment could be repeated hourly as long as the cold laser was not delivering over 10 joules of input to the patient as that is the level that damages DNA.

"Life cannot exist without light. Therefore, if we are sick, injured or in any state of dis-ease we first need to look toward light for answers.[11] The goal of cold laser therapy is to help transform cellular ADP to cellular ATP. ATP is the energy source for cellular function and it takes 400 times more energy for a cell to heal than it does to function normally. The second reason that these specific cold lasers interested me as treatment options for my patients included the fact that I could use some of the generic settings that would help most of my patients immediately. For instance, inflammation and Infection were settings that helped most animal patients. Those that had been prescribed an antibiotic were treated with the infection setting. Inflammation is indicated by five cardinal signs that are well recognized: swelling, heat, redness, pain, and loss of function. There are very few patients that come in to the clinic that aren't experiencing a couple of these symptoms. The lasers work but in animal patients someone must hold the laser and in some cases hold it in direct contact with the patient or at least aim it at the animal for at least three minutes. So this was a limiting factor in treatment of the animal patient. But who was this Rife guy that Dr. Kauffman was so excited about?

In the 20's and 30' Royal Rife developed a way to determine the frequency of soundwave that resonated with single cells (viruses and bacteria) and also non vertebrate parasites that made them explode under the microscope. He was able to help an animal with a spine get rid of these invaders by playing the appropriate frequency near them. He was able to clear 14 of 16 terminal cancer patients of their tumors. Morris Fishbein attempted to purchase the rights to Rife's frequency machine, but he was denied by Rife. Fishbein attacked the theory of healing with frequency in his newspaper columns. Rife's specially built laboratory burned to the ground. Rife was charged with practicing medicine without a license and was dragged through the California courts for two years. Any doctors using the Rife Beam Ray had to cease using it to treat patients for fear of losing their license. A few devices similar to Rife's Beam Ray were developed in foreign countries and were banned in the US by the FDA.[12]

Rife's phanotron was an ingenious instrument that produced the required electric field by means of braking radiation. Instead of emitting EM waves in all directions by means of an antenna, like Hertz did and is usual for broadcasting, his system generated a local beam of EM waves. The destruction of bacteria by resonance was already observable with standard optical microscopes, but Rife was also able to see exploding nanobacteria. Actually, he

---

[11] Website. Dr. Brandon Crawford, DC, FIBFN-CND
[12] Vibrational Medicine. Richard Gerber, MD. 2001

had to persevere for more than a decade to make these tiny microbes visible. He then proved that some of them are present in cancer tissue and that after being cultured, they do also cause cancer. He determined the resonance frequency for targeted destruction of various microbes. These values were confirmed by two collaborators, using different equipment.

Everything, including your body, operates at a vibrating or resonant frequency. Finding the right one with Rife therapy can heal damaged cells. It can also destroy harmful cells and organisms, such as bacteria, viruses, and molds. Rife theory proposes that the frequencies of harmful cells and microorganisms are measurable and recordable. By increasing the resonant frequency, it's possible to raise the vibrations to a level that's intolerable to the target cells. The result is the destruction of harmful cells and improved health. Resonance is a phenomenon which occurs throughout nature. Resonance is the occurrence of a vibrating object causing another object to vibrate a higher amplitude. Resonance happens when the frequency of the initial object's vibration matches the resonant frequency or natural frequency of the second object.[13] Something with resonance has a deep tone or a powerful lasting effect. Resonance is the quality of being "resonant," which can mean "strong and deep in tone" or "having a lasting effect."[14] Living human cells have resonant frequencies – rates at which they will naturally oscillate if the conditions are right. This has been suspected for decades, but researchers have now measured what some of those frequencies are.[15]

Magnetic therapy has been around for a long time. DD Palmer was a magnetic healer before he started practicing Chiropractic. The practice of using magnets in medicine dates to Chinese medical literature at least 2000 years old. Even Paracelsus, one of the most famous doctors in early western medicine, suggests the use of magnets. Using magnets for healing has been popular in Japan since the 1940s. Recently, many athletes have used magnetic wraps on injuries and attest to their success; however, there has been little proof beyond these anecdotes, and no explanation as to how they might work. North and south poles of a magnet have distinct effects. The north pole slows down the processes of life, controls pain, decreases blood pressure and the growth rate of cancer cells, causes retardation of maturation and growth, and increases sensitivity such as intelligence, reflexes, and environmental reaction. The energy created is negative with a counterclockwise electron spin. The south pole strengthens and promotes growth; increases life span, vigor, and vitality; and increases acidity and hyperactivity in the body. It has a clockwise electron expanding spin. While it is not known exactly what effects

---

[13] https://byjus.com/physics/resonance/
[14] https://www.vocabulary.com/dictionary/resonance
[15] https://sageacademyofsound.com/science-of-sound-healing

magnets have on the body, it is known magnetic fields produced by static magnets are different from the electromagnetic fields produced by pulsed electromagnetic field (PEMF) devices, which induce electrical current inside the body.[16]

With PEMF therapy the magnetic fields created by the device travel through and past the skin (including hair or fur, casts, and bandages) to penetrate soft tissue and bones, delivering current throughout the treatment area. This differs from magnets, whose magnetic field can only penetrate a short distance from the magnet and do not cause an electric current to flow. This also differs from electrical devices that deliver electricity directly through paddles or electrodes. These deliver electricity directly to tissue, causing current to flow through a channel of least resistance- which works more like a highway for current to pass through some tissue while leaving the rest unaffected. The electromagnetic field created by PEMF devices reaches all the targeted tissue easily, creating healing effects throughout the treatment area. The fields created by therapeutic magnets generally cannot reach more than an inch or two into the body unlike the depth of PEMF therapy.

Pulsating magnetic fields create increased blood flow to the treated area. The electrically charged ions in the blood will be deflected by the magnetic pole encountered. For example, sodium chloride normally circulates through the blood with zero net charge. As the ions encounter a magnetic field the chloride ions (negative charged) are attracted to the south pole while the sodium ions (positive charged) are detracted. When a series of alternating North-South poles is established over a blood vessel, the positive and negative ions travel side to side in the vessel. The combination of the electromagnetic field, the altered ionic flow pattern and the whirling eddy currents act to dilate the vessels, allowing a greater volume of blood to flow into the area. PEMF also increases oxygen-carrying ability in blood, increases enzyme activity, increases cell division, alters acid-base balance in tissues and alters endocrine activity.

Arthritis and other degenerative joint diseases may benefit from pulsating magnetic therapy. Heart disease, arrhythmia and congestive heart failure patients may benefit from treatment three times weekly with pulsating magnetic fields. Chronic liver, kidney and pancreatic disease patients may benefit from five daily treatments with pulsating magnetic fields. There are many different types of mats on the market, but in its truest sense, it is a mat with electromagnets that are pulsed at a very low, fixed rate. The effects are general, and the output is primarily that of magnetism. The strength of the magnets is low, as well. The units also require direct body contact. A useful device, but with limited capabilities. I

---

[16] https://assisianimalhealth.com/blog/pemf-vs- magnets-whats-the-difference

was very reluctant to get into the PEMF therapy business as I already had two modalities that worked similarly and had fewer limitations.

All of that changed when I was introduced to the QiCoil. A PEMF machine that was programable with over 10,000 frequencies and depending on the unit you choose has the ability to treat an animal within a 10-, 20- or 30-foot radius of the device. Like I said in the beginning;

"You need to purchase a Qi-Coil to ensure your pet's maximum health and well-being."

How we use the Qi-Coil in our practice and household. There are the sudden onset or acute problems and then there are the chronic issues that all creatures develop as they are exposed to more toxins, traumas and emotional roller coasters. Yes, your pet experiences emotional ups and downs just like the human members of the household.

For sudden onset problems and other issues while we are looking for the main problem the treatment should be aimed at decreasing the cardinal signs of inflammation. These signs are swelling, heat, redness, pain, and loss of function. If we can reduce these symptoms as quickly as possible there will be less residual inflammation. I recommend using the Qicoil for 15 minutes, three or four times a day until symptoms are mostly resolved. For chronic issues I would recommend using the settings based on the diagnosis and organs involved in your animals health issues. We let the playlist run during the night and find that our pets with move out of the coils range when they have had enough.

Often we will put the frequency for a homeopathic remedy into the playlist along with the frequencies listed for the condition. Enjoy your QiCoils as they will change the frequency of every member in the family.

Disclaimer: Qi Coils are not approved by the FDA to treat, heal, prevent, or mitigate any disease. The information provided is for general information purposes only and should not be considered a substitute for professional medical advice. Consult a qualified health care professional before using any medical device or products from QiLifeStore.com. Results may vary, and testimonials do not guarantee similar outcomes. By using the products you release Qi Coils and it affiliates from any liability.

Chapter 1: The History of Energy and Frequency Medicine

1.1 Introduction: A Subtle Force Supporting Life

Every generation of healers has sensed that life is more than chemistry and structure. Beneath the visible functions of blood and bone lies a rhythm, a pulse, a resonance that animates living things. From the earliest lodestones of antiquity to the finely tuned electromagnetic devices of today, people have tried to harness this subtle force for healing.

This chapter follows that evolution—from ancient magnetism to D. D. Palmer's magnetic healing in the late nineteenth century, through Tesla's resonant field discoveries, to twentieth-century PEMF and Rife-frequency research. The story ends with modern frequency-controlled systems such as the Qi Coil, which blend chiropractic principles with precision technology to restore coherence in the body's electromagnetic field.

1.2 Ancient Roots: Lodestones, Mesmer, and the Magnetic Imagination
    1.2.1 Lodestones and Early Discovery

Human fascination with magnetism predates written history. Natural magnets—lodestones—were mined and used in ancient Greece, China, and India for navigation, amulets, and early medical practices.[1] Chinese physicians in the Yellow Emperor's Classic of Internal Medicine (ca. 200 BCE) described using magnetized needles to influence energy flow, while the Greek physician Galen recommended magnet stones to draw "morbid humors" from the body.[2]

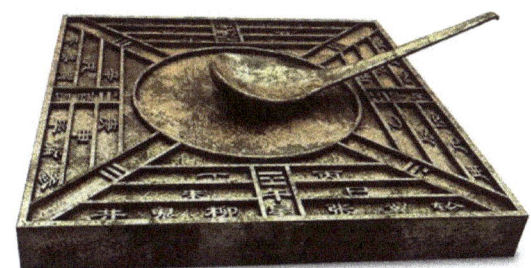

Lodestones represented one of humanity's first encounters with an invisible but palpable force. Though their mechanism was unknown, the ability of a stone to attract metal suggested a hidden current linking matter and motion: a foreshadowing of the field concepts that would later define physics.

An early lodestone compass. The handle of the spoon pointed south as the lodestone balanced on the bronze plate,

    1.2.2 Animal Magnetism and the Mesmer Phenomenon

In the eighteenth century, Franz Anton Mesmer (1734–1815) theorized that living organisms were immersed in a universal fluid he called "animal magnetism".[3] Disease, he claimed, arose when this magnetic flow was obstructed; healing occurred when balance was restored. Mesmer used magnets, gestures, and intention to direct the current, and his dramatic cures captivated Europe.

While royal commissions in France dismissed Mesmer's claims as suggestive rather than physical, his influence endured. The very language of "mesmerism" gave rise to hypnosis, trance therapy, and the continuing idea that consciousness and subtle energy are intertwined. Mesmer planted a seed: that health depends on vibrational harmony.

1.3 The Nineteenth-Century Revolution: From Mystery to Measurement
1.3.1 Faraday, Maxwell, and Electromagnetic Induction

The Industrial Revolution transformed magnetism from magic to mathematics. In 1831, Michael Faraday discovered that a changing magnetic field could induce an electrical current in a conductor—a principle he called "electromagnetic induction".[4] This insight birthed the modern motor, generator, and, eventually, every pulsed-field therapy.

Later, James Clerk Maxwell united electricity and magnetism in his famous equations, showing they were not separate fluids but oscillations in the same field.[5] For medicine, this implied that living tissues—already known to generate bioelectric potentials—might interact dynamically with external fields.

1.3.2 d'Arsonval and the First Magnetic Stimulation

In 1896, French physiologist Jacques Arsène d'Arsonval reported that rapidly changing magnetic fields could induce mild currents in animal tissue without causing pain or burns.[6] His "solenoid chair," essentially a giant coil around the subject's body, produced sensations of warmth, light, and relaxation. D'Arsonval's work prefigured both diathermy and today's pulsed electromagnetic field (PEMF) therapy.

The late 1800s in America were marked by a wide range of alternative healing practices. Conventional medicine relied heavily on bleeding, purging, and harsh chemicals such as mercury. Many people sought gentler, non-drug therapies. This environment allowed movements like homeopathy, osteopathy, hydropathy, and magnetic healing to flourish. Spiritualism and the idea that unseen forces influenced health and disease were widely discussed.[7] Palmer, an inquisitive man who had studied anatomy, physiology, and natural philosophy, was drawn to these currents of thought.

1.4 Magnetism Meets Medicine: 1900–1930
1.4.1 D. D. Palmer and Magnetic Healing

D.D. Palmer was a man of many trades before becoming a healer. He farmed, kept bees, and worked in a variety of occupations. Around 1886 he turned his full attention to magnetic healing, opening an office in Davenport. He advertised himself as a "magnetic healer," offering to treat without drugs or surgery.[8] His records show that he attracted a steady clientele, many of whom had chronic conditions that conventional medicine had failed to help.

Palmer's approach combined careful observation, palpation, and his own theories about the flow of vital force. He was known to place his hands directly on areas of complaint and concentrate on "pouring" his magnetic energy into the patient. At the same time, he studied the relationship between the nervous system and health, gradually developing a more mechanical explanation for why patients improved under his care.[9] Although Palmer's magnetic healing practice was successful, he was not satisfied with vague explanations. He sought a more precise cause-and-effect understanding of health and disease. His curiosity led him to study the spine, the nervous system, and the mechanics of the body. He noticed that many patients had tender areas or palpable irregularities in the spine, and that working with these areas seemed to produce consistent results.

This line of inquiry culminated in September 1895 when Palmer adjusted Harvey Lillard, a janitor who had been deaf for 17 years. According to Palmer, he felt a misaligned vertebra in Lillard's back, adjusted it, and Lillard's hearing improved.[10] Palmer concluded that restoring normal alignment of the spine could free the nervous system from interference, allowing the body's natural healing power to flow. Chiropractic was born. His shift from magnets to manual adjustment did not abandon the energetic worldview; it refined it. Chiropractic, from its inception, was rooted in the belief that tone and vibration govern health.

1.4.2 Nikola Tesla and Resonant Energy

At the same time, Nikola Tesla was electrifying the world—literally and philosophically. His inventions in alternating current and rotating magnetic fields proved that oscillating energy could travel through space without wires.[11] Tesla's experiments with high-frequency currents and vacuum tubes inspired early "violet-ray" and coil-based healing devices. He believed every organism had a resonant frequency and that illness reflected disharmony in that resonance.

1.4.3 Early Electrotherapy and Diathermy

By the early twentieth century, electrotherapy had entered mainstream medicine. Physicians used high-frequency current—diathermy—to warm tissues, reduce pain, and increase circulation.[12] Although many commercial devices were poorly regulated and over-promised miraculous cures, legitimate research established that pulsed currents could influence physiology beyond simple heating.

1.5 Between Science and Speculation: 1930–1960
1.5.1 Royal Rife and Frequency-Specific Medicine

In the 20's and 30' Royal Rife developed a way to determine the frequency of soundwave that resonated with single cells (viruses and bacteria) and also non vertebrate parasites that made them explode under the microscope. He was able to help an animal with a spine get rid of these invaders by playing the appropriate frequency near them. He was able to clear 14 of 16 terminal cancer patients of their tumors. Morris Fishbein attempted to purchase the rights to Rife's frequency machine, but he was denied by Rife. Fishbein attacked the theory of healing with frequency in his newspaper columns. Rife's specially built laboratory burned to the ground. Rife was charged with practicing medicine without a license and was dragged through the California courts for two years. Any doctors using the Rife Beam Ray had to cease using it to treat patients for fear of losing their license. A few devices similar to Rife's Beam Ray were developed in foreign countries and were banned in the US by the FDA.[13]

Rife's Phanotron was an ingenious instrument that produced the required electric field by means of braking radiation. Instead of emitting EM waves in all directions by means of an antenna, like Hertz did and is usual for broadcasting, his system generated a local beam of EM waves. The destruction of bacteria by resonance was already observable with standard optical microscopes, but Rife was also able to see exploding nanobacteria. Actually, he had to persevere for more than a decade to make these tiny microbes visible. He then proved that some of them are present in cancer tissue and that after being cultured, they do also cause cancer. He determined the resonance frequency for targeted destruction of various microbes. These values were confirmed by two collaborators, using different equipment.

Everything, including your dog's body, operates at a vibrating or resonant frequency. Finding the right one with Rife therapy can heal damaged cells. It can also destroy harmful cells and organisms, such as bacteria, viruses, and molds. Rife theory proposes that the frequencies of harmful cells and microorganisms are measurable and recordable. By increasing the resonant frequency, it's possible to raise the vibrations to a level that's intolerable to the target cells. The result is the destruction of harmful cells and improved health. Resonance is a phenomenon which occurs throughout nature. Resonance is the occurrence of a vibrating object causing another object to vibrate a higher amplitude. Resonance happens when the frequency of the initial object's vibration matches the resonant frequency or natural frequency of the second object.[14] Something with resonance has a deep tone or a powerful lasting effect. Resonance is the quality of being "resonant," which can mean "strong and deep in tone" or "having a lasting effect."[15] Living human cells have resonant frequencies – rates at which they will naturally oscillate if the conditions are right. This has been suspected for decades, but researchers have now measured what some of those frequencies are.[16]

Rife introduced the crucial idea that specific frequencies might exert selective biological effects.

1.5.2 Lakhovsky and the Multiwave Oscillator

Around the same period, Georges Lakhovsky developed the multiwave oscillator, which generated a broad spectrum of electromagnetic frequencies intended to "re-tune" cells.[17] He theorized that living cells act as tiny oscillators; disease begins when their natural vibration weakens. Lakhovsky's work, though marginalized after World War II, foreshadowed the concept of bioresonance.

1.5.3 Transition Toward Pulsed Fields

Post-war research began distinguishing between continuous (static) fields and pulsed or time-varying ones. Studies showed that intermittent pulses could stimulate bone and nerve tissue regeneration more effectively than steady exposure.[18] This discovery marked the birth of modern PEMF therapy.

1.6 The Biomedical Era: 1960–2000
1.6.1 C. Andrew Bassett and Orthopedic Breakthroughs

Orthopedic surgeon C. Andrew Bassett at Columbia University demonstrated that low-frequency pulsed electromagnetic fields could accelerate the healing of non-union fractures.[19] In 1979, the U.S. Food and Drug Administration cleared the first PEMF bone-growth stimulator—a milestone validating electromedicine in clinical practice.

1.6.2 Soviet and NASA Research

During the Cold War, Soviet scientists explored PEMF for pain, circulation, and athletic recovery. Their protocols eventually informed space-medicine programs in both East and West. NASA later employed weak pulsed fields to counteract bone and muscle loss in astronauts.[20] A 2003 NASA report by Thomas Goodwin described enhanced cellular regeneration in tissue cultures exposed to specific electromagnetic patterns.[21]

1.6.3 Neuroscience Applications: Transcranial Magnetic Stimulation

In 1985, Anthony Barker introduced Transcranial Magnetic Stimulation (TMS), showing that brief magnetic pulses could depolarize neurons through the skull.[22] TMS became an FDA-approved treatment for depression and opened new understanding of electromagnetic influence on the nervous system—precisely the domain chiropractors seek to balance.

1.6.4 Critique and Consolidation

Skeptics argued that many PEMF studies lacked rigorous controls. Yet meta-analyses through the 1990s showed consistent benefits for pain and bone repair.[23] The field matured from experimental curiosity to recognized adjunct therapy, albeit still misunderstood by conventional medicine.

1.7 From Static Magnets to Dynamic Resonance

Static magnets enjoyed consumer popularity in the late twentieth century—bracelets, shoe inserts, mattress pads—but produced inconsistent clinical results.[24] Pulsed fields, by contrast, induced measurable electrical changes in tissue. They resonated.

Resonance distinguishes Qi Coil–style technology from inert magnet products. Frequency, waveform, and timing can entrain cellular oscillations, affecting ion transport, ATP synthesis, and nitric-oxide signaling.[25] The conversation has shifted from magnetism as force to resonance as communication.

Comparison of Static vs. Pulsed Magnetic Field Effects

Static magnetic field	Pulsed magnetic field
Constant	Oscillating
• No signal	• Signal

1.8 Digital Frequency Medicine and the Qi Coil Lineage
1.8.1 Microelectronics and Waveform Control

With the rise of microprocessors, frequency devices became precise and programmable. Software now modulates amplitude, duty cycle, and harmonic layering, allowing practitioners to design specific healing environments. Libraries of "frequency sets" mirror Rife's concept but are grounded in contemporary biofeedback data.

1.8.2 Field Geometry and the Toroid Advantage

Modern designers learned that coil geometry shapes biological response. A toroidal coil—essentially a doughnut shape—confines the magnetic flux within a closed loop, minimizing stray radiation while creating a concentrated, penetrating field. Qi Coil employs this geometry to surround the user in a balanced vortex of energy rather than a directional beam.

The design echoes Tesla's fascination with rotating fields: energy circulating harmoniously instead of linearly.[26]

1.8.3 App-Driven Accessibility

Qi Coil systems integrate Bluetooth and smartphone apps, delivering curated frequency programs: pain relief, regeneration, focus, emotional balance. The convenience of digital control democratizes what once required laboratory equipment. Users can select, layer, or loop frequencies, aligning sessions with chiropractic visits, meditation, or sleep.

1.8.4 Safety and Standardization

PEMF exposure guidelines from WHO and IEC inform modern device limits. Qi Coil's output remains well below occupational exposure thresholds, ensuring comfort even during long sessions.[27] Its non-contact design eliminates current conduction risk, distinguishing it from electrode-based electrotherapy.

1.9 Philosophical Continuities: Energy and Innate Intelligence

Throughout history, the underlying philosophy has remained remarkably constant:

Era	Term	Core Idea
Ancient	Vital breath, Qi, Prana	Life arises from Universal energy flow.
Mesmer (18th century)	Animal Magnetism	Illness equals blockage of subtle current.
Palmer (19th century)	Innate Intelligence	Nerve interference disturbs expression.
Tesla (20th century)	Resonance and frequency	Everything vibrates, harmony equals health.
PEMF and Qi Coil (21st century)	Coherent biofield modulation	Tuned fields restore systemic balance

Table 1. Magnetic Energy Evolution

Both chiropractic and frequency medicine view the organism as a self-organizing field seeking balance. The chiropractor adjusts the structure to free the nerve flow; the frequency practitioner adjusts the field to free the energetic flow. In truth, these are the same act performed on different layers of the same system.

Magnetic healing was the seedbed in which D.D. Palmer's ideas about health took root. While chiropractic would ultimately diverge from its magnetic origins, the practice gave Palmer the experience, the patients, and the philosophical framework to develop a new system of healing. By blending the hands-on, drugless ethos of magnetic healing with a focus on anatomy and nerve function, Palmer created chiropractic; a discipline that has endured long after magnetic healing faded from the mainstream. It is a drugless healing philosophy as magnetic healing convinced Palmer that the body could heal itself without drugs or surgery. Chiropractic maintained this core principle. He continued the hands-on therapy that he had practiced before Harvey Lillard as this gave Palmer the tactile skills and confidence to work physically with patients, a direct precursor to spinal adjusting.

Chiropractic was based on vitalism and Innate Intelligence; the idea that unseen forces or energies governed health was reinterpreted by Palmer into the chiropractic concept of Innate Intelligence, the body's inborn wisdom that coordinates healing.[28] As with magnetic healing, chiropractic emphasized listening to patients, providing individualized care, and offering hope where medicine often failed.

Yet, even as chiropractic grew, the influence of magnetic healing lingered. Early chiropractic writings often spoke of nerve force and the body's innate power in ways reminiscent of magnetic concepts.[29] The transition from magnetic healer to chiropractor reflects both Palmer's visionary creativity and his desire to place healing on a more scientific foundation.

1.10 Convergence with Chiropractic Care

When D. D. Palmer spoke of "tone," he referred not merely to muscle tension but to the vibrational quality of living tissue. Frequency medicine literalizes that metaphor. Pulsed electromagnetic fields can prime the nervous system, relax hypertonic muscles, and enhance communication before an adjustment; then stabilize tissues afterward.

Qi Coil technology, in this sense, is the natural heir to chiropractic philosophy. It allows practitioners to:
> Prepare the patient or animal with pre-adjustment frequency entrainment.
> Adjust with greater ease and precision due to relaxed musculature.
> Integrate the change post-adjustment through regenerative frequency sets.

Where Palmer used the term Universal Intelligence, today's clinician might speak of quantum coherence. Both describe the same phenomenon: organized energy expressing itself through matter.

1.11 Conclusion: The Legacy Continues

From Mesmer's salons to NASA's laboratories, the history of energy medicine is the story of humankind's desire to work with nature's forces rather than against them. Each generation refines the tools but pursues the same goal, harmony.

Modern devices like the Qi Coil encapsulate centuries of exploration in one elegant system: a toroidal conductor guided by software, bridging physics and philosophy. They stand as living proof that the healing currents D. D. Palmer sensed under his hands are real, measurable, and now tunable.

As chiropractic care evolves to embrace frequency technologies, the ancient art of balancing life's magnetic rhythms finds its modern expression, not as mysticism, but as measurable resonance.

1. Edward R. Lippincott, The Lodestone and Its Mysteries (London: Routledge, 1998), 12–15.
2. Huang Di Nei Jing, trans. Ilza Veith (Berkeley: University of California Press, 1949), 74.
3. Franz A. Mesmer, Mémoire sur la découverte du magnétisme animal (Paris: Didot, 1779).
4. Michael Faraday, Experimental Researches in Electricity, vol. 1 (London: Taylor, 1839).
5. James Clerk Maxwell, A Treatise on Electricity and Magnetism (Oxford: Clarendon, 1873).
6. J. A. d'Arsonval, "Action Physiologique des Courants Alternatifs," Comptes Rendus de l'Académie des Sciences 123 (1896): 283–85.
7. Gevitz, N. (1988). Other Healers: Unorthodox Medicine in America. Johns Hopkins University Press.
8. Palmer, D. D. (1910/1966). The Chiropractor's Adjuster: The Science, Art and Philosophy of Chiropractic. Portland, OR: Portland Printing House / reprint by National Chiropractic Mutual Insurance Co.
9. Keating, J. C. (1995). B.J. of Davenport: The Early Years of Chiropractic. Davenport, IA: Association for the History of Chiropractic.
10. Palmer, D. D. (1910/1966). The Chiropractor's Adjuster: The Science, Art and Philosophy of Chiropractic. Portland, OR: Portland Printing House / reprint by National Chiropractic Mutual Insurance Co.
11. Nikola Tesla, "The Problem of Increasing Human Energy," Century Magazine (1900): 175–211.
12. Karl F. Nagelschmidt, Diathermy and Short-Wave Therapy (Berlin: Springer, 1913).
13. Vibrational Medicine. Richard Gerber, MD. 2001
14. https://byjus.com/physics/resonance/
15. https://www.vocabulary.com/dictionary/resonance
16. https://sageacademyofsound.com/science-of-sound-healing
17. Georges Lakhovsky, The Secret of Life (New York: New Century, 1939).
18. C. Andrew Bassett et al., "Effects of Pulsing Electromagnetic Fields on Bone Repair," Journal of Bone and Joint Surgery 58-A (1976): 993–1003.
19. Ibid.
20. V. Novikova, "PEMF Therapy in Soviet Sports Medicine," Bioelectromagnetics 5 (1984): 201–08.
21. Thomas Goodwin, "Physiological Effects of Electromagnetic Fields on Tissue Repair," NASA Technical Report CR-2003-212054 (Houston: NASA, 2003).
22. A. T. Barker et al., "Non-invasive Magnetic Stimulation of Human Motor Cortex," The Lancet 1 (1985): 1106–07.
23. Mark Pollack, "Meta-Analysis of PEMF in Pain and Healing," Clinical Orthopedics (1998): 25–33.
24. Richard P. Ernst, "Static Magnet Therapy: Review of Evidence," Complementary Therapies in Medicine 11 (2003): 95–101.

25. W. Markov and M. Colbert, "Magnetic Field Therapy: A Review," Electromagnetic Biology and Medicine (2001): 17–36.
26. Nikola Tesla, Colorado Springs Notes, 1899–1900 (New York: Nolit, 1978).
27. World Health Organization, Environmental Health Criteria 232: Static Fields (Geneva: WHO, 2006).
28. Wardwell, W. I. (1992). Chiropractic: History and Evolution of a New Profession. Mosby-Year Book.
29. Keating, J. C. (1997). History of Chiropractic: A Primer. Association for the History of Chiropractic.

Chapter 2: Chiropractic and Energy — Parallel Philosophies

2.1 Introduction: Two Languages, One Law

Chiropractic and energy medicine are two expressions of a single truth: life is organized energy flowing through matter. The chiropractor speaks of Innate Intelligence and the nervous system; the energy physician speaks of vibration, resonance, and coherence. Each describes the same process—the transmission of information that maintains the harmony of living systems. Whether that information travels along a spinal nerve or a magnetic waveform, its purpose is identical: to coordinate the body's self-healing potential.

Animal chiropractic brings this principle into sharp relief because it must cross species lines. The same universal laws that govern human neuro-energetics also shape the equine spinal column, the canine limb reflex, and the bovine rumen nerve plexus. Understanding these parallels allows the practitioner to perceive the unity beneath the diversity of form.

2.2 The Vitalistic Foundations of Chiropractic
    2.2.1 D. D. Palmer and the Magnetic Origins

When we look at the origins of chiropractic, it is easy to focus on the dramatic moment in 1895 when Daniel David Palmer, a Canadian-born healer living in Davenport, Iowa, performed what he later called the first chiropractic adjustment on Harvey Lillard. Yet to understand the philosophy and practice that gave rise to chiropractic, we must step back into Palmer's earlier career. Before chiropractic, D.D. Palmer was a practitioner of what was then called magnetic healing. This phase of his life, stretching from the mid-1880s through the early 1890s, set the stage for the system of spinal adjustments and innate intelligence that would later become his lasting legacy.

When D. D. Palmer performed the first chiropractic adjustment in 1895, he was already a magnetic healer by trade.[1] He believed disease resulted from "displacement of vital energy" and that realignment of the body's structure restored the flow of this energy through the nerves. His early notebooks mention polarities, currents, and vibrations, terms drawn as much from physics as from metaphysics. Chiropractic thus began not as a rejection of energetic concepts but as their refinement into anatomical specificity.

    2.2.2 B. J. Palmer and the Nerve as Conductor

Palmer's son, Bartlett Joshua (B. J.) Palmer, reframed the spinal column as an antenna for Innate Intelligence. He compared the vertebrae to the tuning dials of a radio: when subluxated, the body receives "static" instead of clear signal.[2] His writings anticipate modern bioresonance theory, suggesting that neural tissue both transmits and receives vibrational information. B. J.'s torque-release and HIO (Hole-in-One) techniques aimed to remove interference at the atlas, restoring global harmony throughout the system.

2.2.3 Stephenson's Principles and the Law of Tone

In 1927, Ralph Stephenson codified Palmer's philosophy in The Chiropractic Textbook, listing thirty-three principles.[3] Among them, Principle No. 9 defines tone as "the normal degree of nerve tension" and the expression of Innate Intelligence through matter. To Stephenson, tone was both a mechanical and vibrational state, a bridge concept linking biology to physics. This notion of tone provides the conceptual hinge connecting chiropractic to modern frequency therapy.

2.3 Innate Intelligence and Universal Resonance
2.3.1 The Organizing Field

Chiropractic posits that a non-material intelligence animates living systems. In modern language, this corresponds to the idea of an organizing field—what biophysicist Rupert Sheldrake later termed morphogenetic fields[4] and what contemporary quantum biologists describe as biofields. These models propose that biological order arises from informational patterns carried by electromagnetic and scalar interactions.

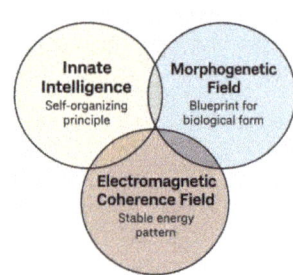

Diagram 2: Interconnected Concepts Diagram

2.3.2 Neuro-Energetic Correlates

From a physiological standpoint, the nervous system translates energetic potential into biological command. Every neuron maintains a transmembrane voltage of roughly –70 mV; depolarization propagates signals as oscillating electrical waves. These oscillations generate measurable magnetic fields (magnetoencephalography and magnetocardiography record them daily). Thus, the living body is literally an electromagnetic instrument, and subluxation can be understood as interference in wave transmission.

2.3.3 Vibration as the Common Denominator

D. D. Palmer once wrote, "Life is a condition of tone." Modern physics would restate this: life is a condition of vibration. Whether one speaks of Qi, Prana, or Innate, the operative element is frequency. Healthy tissue vibrates in coherent patterns; diseased tissue vibrates chaotically. Adjustment and frequency therapy both seek to re-establish coherence.

2.4 Comparative Neuro-Energetic Physiology

Because animal chiropractors work across species, they witness directly how Innate Intelligence expresses through diverse neural architectures. Despite anatomical differences, the principles of flow, adaptation, and vibrational harmony remain constant.

2.4.1 Structural Overview

Species	Vertebral Formula	Spinal Cord Terminates	Unique Adaptations
Canine	7 C / 13 T / 7 L / 3 S / 20 Ca	L6-L7	Highly mobile cervical spine for sensory orientation; strong sympathetic tone.
Equine	7 C / 18 T / 6 L / 5 S / 18 Ca	S1-S2	Massive epaxial musculature; limited lateral flexion; strong parasympathetic vagal control of gut.
Bovine	7 C / 13 T / 6 L / 5 S / 19 Ca	S1	Heavy rumen innervation via dorsal and ventral vagal trunks; weight-bearing thoracic rigidity.
Human	7 C / 12 T / 5 L / 5 S / 3 Ca	L1-L2	Upright posture; sacral plexus specialized for bipedal balance.

Table 2: Comparative vertebral segmentation among mammals.

Despite differences, all mammals share the same fundamental neuro-energetic template: ascending sensory pathways, descending motor pathways, and autonomic loops coordinating viscera and behavior. The subluxation complex; mechanical, neurological, and energetic; disturbs this template by altering afferent input and efferent output.

2.4.2 Autonomic Regulation and Energy Flow

The sympathetic chain ganglia function as step-down transformers, modulating energy distribution throughout the body. Excess sympathetic tone corresponds to chronic "fight-or-flight" energy stagnation, while parasympathetic dominance fosters repair. Chiropractic adjustment acts as a reset switch, re-balancing these oscillations.[5] In animals, this is often visible as a sigh, ear flick, or muscle fasciculation immediately post-adjustment.

Parameter	Before Adjustment	After Adjustment	Physiologic Interpretation
Sympathetic Tone	Elevated (↑ HR, ↑ RR, muscle tension, vigilance)	Reduced to normal (HR and RR stabilize, muscles relax)	Indicates decreased "fight-or-flight" activity.
Parasympathetic Tone	↓ Digestive function and immune response	Enhanced (improved) digestion, calm demeanor, normalized salivation	Reflects activation of "rest-and-digest" processes.
Heart Rate Variability (HRV)	Low (reduced adaptability to stress)	Increased (improved autonomic balance and resilience)	Higher HRV = greater adaptability and nervous system coherence.
Postural Reflexes	Compensatory muscle guarding or imbalance	Balanced postural tone, improved weight distribution	Suggests restored proprioceptive input and spinal alignment.
Behavior / Affect	Anxious, reactive, or restless	Calm, alert, responsive	Behavioral markers of nervous system balance
Overall Autonomic State	Sympathetic dominance	Dynamic equilibrium (parasympathetic recovery)	Represents improved homeostatic regulation and energy efficiency.

Table 3: Autonomic nervous-system balance before and after adjustment.

2.4.3 Species-Specific Expressions of Subluxation

Canine: Rapid acceleration, twisting, and play lead to recurrent thoracolumbar fixations. Energetically, dogs exhibit acute sympathetic bursts followed by sudden fatigue; analogous to "spiking then crashing" in human stress physiology.

Equine: Long lever arms of the neck and lumbar spine make horses prone to kinetic chain distortions. Their large energy fields and herd sensitivity amplify subtle vibrational cues; an anxious handler's tone often mirrors in the horse's musculature.

Bovine: Limited spinal motion and heavy visceral load create low-grade fixations that subtly alter vagal tone, influencing digestion and milk yield. Adjustments often normalize rumen motility; an energetic as well as mechanical correction.

2.5 The Bridge Between Physics and Physiology
2.5.1 Piezoelectric and Electromagnetic Properties of Tissue

Collagen, bone, and fascia exhibit piezoelectricity—the ability to generate electrical charge when mechanically stressed.[6] Each chiropractic adjustment therefore sends a micro-current pulse through the connective matrix, reinforcing the concept that mechanical force translates into electromagnetic signaling. This "biomechanical resonance" provides the physiological substrate for the philosophical claim that "structure affects function."

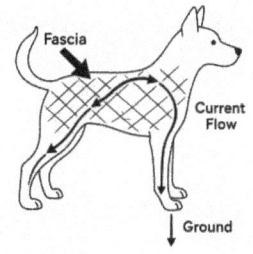

2.5.2 Fascia as an Energetic Continuum

Recent veterinary fascial research describes a continuous network linking muscle spindles, visceral ligaments, and periosteum.[7] This network conducts not only mechanical tension but also biophotonic and electromagnetic information. When restricted, it behaves like a kinked fiber-optic cable—scattering light instead of transmitting it coherently. Chiropractic adjustments and gentle motion restore linearity, re-establishing clear energetic communication.

Diagram 3: Fascia works as a conductive lattice; stress-induced current flow is slowed down.

2.5.3 The Quantum Perspective

Quantum biology suggests that electrons within protein structures may tunnel or transfer energy coherently over nanometer distances.[8] Enzyme catalysis, mitochondrial respiration, and even olfaction display quantum coherence. Thus, life's processes depend on maintaining resonance at scales far smaller than nerves. The vertebral subluxation, by altering tissue tension and hydration, may disturb these quantum couplings, producing systemic disorganization.

2.5.4 Chiropractic as Resonance Restoration

From this perspective, an adjustment is not merely a joint manipulation; it is an act of re-tuning. The high-velocity, low-amplitude thrust sends a waveform through the musculoskeletal-neural continuum, briefly interrupting maladaptive oscillations and allowing Innate Intelligence to re-establish phase coherence. The audible cavitation marks the release of both mechanical and vibrational interference. In animals, where verbal feedback is absent, post-adjustment behavioral calm confirms the energetic reset.

2.6 Comparative Manifestations of Energy Imbalance
2.6.1 Behavioral and Postural Indicators

Every species communicates energetic disharmony differently. Veterinarians and animal chiropractors learn to read these non-verbal cues as reflections of neuro-energetic imbalance.

Species	Common Behavioral Signs	Probable Neurological / Energetic Correlate
Canine	Reluctance to jump, circling before lying down, excessive licking of joints	Thoracolumbar fixation → sympathetic overdrive
Equine	Head tossing, tail swishing, shortened stride, avoidance of girth	Cervical or sacroiliac restriction → disrupted vagal tone
Bovine	Uneven weight-bearing, kicking during milking, decreased feed intake	Lumbosacral fixation → altered splanchnic nerve flow

Table 4: Behavioral correlates of subluxation and energy imbalance.

A dog that chronically "hunches" after play, or a horse that resists flexion to one side, is not merely demonstrating musculoskeletal pain but a systemic loss of resonance. The nervous system, deprived of coherent afferent feedback, oscillates erratically. Adjustment restores rhythm—the physiological expression of harmony.

2.6.2 Somato-Visceral Relationships

Chiropractic recognizes that spinal interference affects visceral organs via the autonomic nervous system. Veterinary research confirms parallel patterns across species: gastric motility, heart rate variability, and immune modulation all change in response to spinal manipulation.[9] Energetically, these represent the body's attempt to synchronize internal oscillators—heart, gut, and cortex—into a unified beat.

2.7 The Animal as a Vibrational Organism
2.7.1 Field Perception and Herd Coherence

Animals live immersed in energy exchange. Horses synchronize heart rhythms within herds; dogs entrain to human emotional states through subtle electromagnetic coupling.[10] Studies using heart-rate variability demonstrate that calm handlers induce parasympathetic dominance in their animals—a measurable energetic rapport.[11] The animal chiropractor, entering this field consciously, becomes part of the therapeutic resonance system.

2.7.2 Sensory Extensions of Energy Awareness

Equine vibrissae detect minute electrical and mechanical vibrations.

Canine olfaction converts molecular vibration into neural signal—an energy translation process at the quantum level.

Avian magnetoreception utilizes cryptochrome photopigments sensitive to Earth's magnetic field, illustrating that biological life is magnetically tuned.[12]

When chiropractic correction normalizes spinal alignment, it likely improves not only biomechanical function but also these subtle sensory channels of energetic perception.

2.7.3 Emotional Resonance

Animals express emotion somatically. A stressed horse tightens the poll and withers; a fearful dog tucks the tail and flexes the lumbar spine. These postures alter neural firing, blood flow, and field emission. Restoring alignment releases not only physical tension but the stored vibrational imprint of emotion—a process familiar to practitioners who observe spontaneous sighs, tremors, or licking during adjustment.

2.8 Philosophical Parallels with Modern Energy Technologies
2.8.1 Chiropractic and Frequency Coherence

Chiropractic and modern frequency technologies such as PEMF or Qi Coil are not competitors; they are partners in the same vibrational orchestra. Both operate on the law that organized energy directs organized matter. An adjustment re-establishes conduction through the nervous system; a frequency field re-establishes coherence through the extracellular matrix. Together they express the axiom: as above, so below—structure and field reflecting one another.

2.8.2 The Qi Coil as Modern Expression of Innate Flow

Where D. D. Palmer used his hands as conductors of magnetic intent, Qi Coil uses a toroidal field to broadcast coherent frequency patterns. The device functions as an external extension of the chiropractor's intention. It resonates with Principle No. 24 of Stephenson's text—"The limits of adaptation are determined by the limitations of matter." By providing an energetic environment conducive to adaptation, Qi Coil widens those limits without violating the law of time and natural healing.

2.8.3 The Role of Intention and Consciousness

Quantum biophysics increasingly supports the idea that observer intention influences field coherence.[13] Chiropractic philosophy anticipated this by emphasizing the practitioner's mental state during adjustment. In animal work, calm focus and compassionate intention translate directly into measurable physiological calm in patients. The Qi Coil, when used within this mindful framework, becomes an amplifier of coherent consciousness.

2.9 Integrative Philosophy for the Veterinary Chiropractor

2.9.1 Bridging Objective Science and Subjective Perception

Veterinary professionals trained in anatomy and pathology often struggle to articulate energetic phenomena within biomedical language. The bridge lies in recognizing that electromagnetic descriptions and vitalistic descriptions refer to the same events at different scales. Depolarization potential equals nerve impulse equals vibrational communication. Using this translation, chiropractors and veterinarians can converse without abandoning their respective epistemologies.

2.9.2 Ethical and Professional Integration

Ethically, integration demands evidence-informed use of all modalities. Frequency therapy must complement, not replace, hands-on evaluation and conventional medicine. When applied responsibly, it enhances welfare by reducing reliance on pharmaceuticals and improving recovery. This alignment with One-Health principles situates chiropractic energy work within a larger ecological ethic.

2.9.3 Educational Implications

Training programs for animal chiropractors should include modules on bioenergetics, tissue conductivity, and quantum physiology, allowing future practitioners to understand frequency tools scientifically rather than mystically. As research expands, continuing education can document physiological markers—heart-rate variability, thermography, biophoton emission—that quantify energetic change post-adjustment.

2.10 Conclusion: Harmony Across Species and Systems

In every nervous system—canine, equine, bovine, or human—life expresses through vibration. Chiropractic and energy medicine are complementary dialects of that universal language. The spinal adjustment is a focused act of resonance; the electromagnetic field is its environmental chorus.

The animal chiropractor, standing between structure and field, translates Innate Intelligence into tangible physiology. Whether by the gentle thrust of an atlas adjustment or the whisper of a toroidal pulse from a Qi Coil, the intention is identical: to restore the melody of life where noise has intruded.

In recognizing this, practitioners honor both the founders who spoke of tone and the modern scientists who speak of frequency. The names change; the principle endures. Life is vibration seeking coherence, and healing is the return of harmony.

1. D. D. Palmer, The Chiropractor's Adjuster (Davenport: Palmer College, 1910).
2. B. J. Palmer, The Bigness of the Fellow Within (Davenport: Palmer School of Chiropractic, 1949), 73–78.
3. Ralph W. Stephenson, The Chiropractic Textbook (Davenport: Palmer School of Chiropractic, 1927).
4. Rupert Sheldrake, A New Science of Life: The Hypothesis of Formative Causation (London: Blond & Briggs, 1981).
5. I. P. Pavlov, The Work of the Digestive Glands, 2nd ed. (London: Charles Griffin, 1910).
6. Albert Szent-Györgyi, "Electronic Biology and Cancer," Science 161 (1968): 988–990.
7. Carla Stecco et al., "Fascial Continuity in Veterinary Anatomy," Journal of Equine Veterinary Science 78 (2019): 27–34.
8. John Joe McFadden, "Quantum Evolution of Biological Systems," Trends in Biochemical Sciences 35 (2010): 1–9.
9. Heidi K. Buerger and Shannon J. Green, "Visceral Responses to Spinal Manipulation in the Horse," Veterinary Clinics of North America: Equine Practice 36 (2020): 203–216.
10. Rollin McCraty et al., "The Energetic Heart: Bioelectromagnetic Communication Within and Between People," HeartMath Research Center Technical Report (1998).
11. Ellen Gehrke and Ann Baldwin, "The Horse–Human Heart Connection: The Concept of Heart Coherence," Journal of Equine Veterinary Science 32 (2012): 596–603.
12. Thorsten Ritz et al., "Magnetoreception and Its Use in Animal Navigation," Nature 429 (2004): 177–180.
13. Dean Radin, Entangled Minds: Extrasensory Experiences in a Quantum Reality (New York: Simon & Schuster, 2006).

Chapter 3: The Science of Resonance and Cellular Communication

3.1 Introduction: Life as Organized Vibration

From the cellular level to the coordination of an entire herd, life expresses itself as a series of oscillations. Every heartbeat, breath, neuronal impulse, and muscular contraction occurs in rhythm, forming a nested hierarchy of resonant events that collectively define vitality. Resonance, in its simplest sense, is the capacity of one system to influence another through frequency matching. When two tuning forks vibrate at identical tones, the second begins to hum sympathetically; so too does one biological oscillator entrain another.[1]

In chiropractic and in modern frequency medicine, resonance provides the physical explanation for what D. D. Palmer called tone. Tone is not merely muscular tension but the vibrational state of living tissue. When tone is balanced, energy flows without distortion and the nervous system communicates coherently with every organ and cell. When tone is lost or exaggerated, resonance is replaced by dissonance—what we recognize clinically as dysfunction.

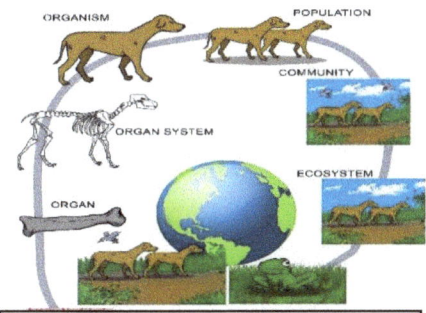

Diagram 4: Nested hierarchy of oscillations from molecule → cell → organ → organism → herd.

Veterinary chiropractic encounters resonance daily. An anxious horse that resists the halter, a dog trembling on the table, or a cow shifting weight unevenly all display disrupted rhythm at behavioral and cellular levels. After adjustment, the breathing slows, muscle tone softens, and the practitioner feels a subtle harmonic "settling." Such observations, repeated across species, reveal that health is coherence—disease, incoherence.

The field of biophysics now validates this ancient intuition. Molecules within living cells oscillate at characteristic frequencies determined by their mass, bonding, and surrounding electromagnetic environment.[2] Proteins fold and unfold rhythmically; DNA emits measurable photonic pulses; mitochondria release electrons in beat-like sequences through their respiratory chains.[3] Life is music played in molecular time.

Resonance becomes both metaphor and mechanism: metaphor, because it evokes harmony and synchronization; mechanism, because entrainment among oscillators transmits information faster than chemical diffusion. When a chiropractic adjustment corrects a subluxation, it re-establishes structural alignment that allows electrical and vibrational signals to travel unimpeded. When a Qi Coil delivers a coherent magnetic field, it similarly invites disordered systems to retune. In both cases, the healer is restoring rhythm.

3.2 Cellular Bioelectricity and Communication
3.2.1 The Cell as an Electrical Organism

Every living cell is an electrical entity. Its membrane separates two ionically distinct fluids: a negatively charged cytoplasm and a positively charged extracellular milieu. This separation creates a potential difference of roughly –70 mV in mammals, though it varies among species and tissues.[4] Ion channels act as transistors, opening and closing in millisecond cycles that constitute the cell's electrical "language." The result is a constant hum of oscillating voltage; the first level of biological resonance.

In neural tissue these oscillations manifest as action potentials; in cardiac muscle as rhythmic depolarization; in secretory cells as calcium-wave bursts that trigger enzyme release. Because the same ions—sodium, potassium, calcium, and chloride—carry charge in all species, the fundamental electrical vocabulary of life is universal. What differs is tempo: the resting potential of equine myocytes fluctuates more slowly than that of canines, matching each species' metabolic rate.[5]

3.2.2 Frequency Coding and Information Transfer

Cells do not simply fire or remain silent; they encode information in frequency. Rapid pulse trains signal urgency, while slower oscillations convey maintenance or repair. The nervous system uses this principle to coordinate thousands of processes simultaneously. For example, a canine's motor neurons firing at 40 Hz maintain postural tone, whereas bursts above 100 Hz trigger explosive movement.[6] Similar frequency-dependent modulation appears in equine gut peristalsis and bovine cardiac rhythm.

Diagram 5: Schematic of a mammalian cell showing ion gradients and oscillating membrane potential.

This insight parallels chiropractic philosophy: interference—whether mechanical or electrical; alters the frequency code. A compressed spinal segment changes the pattern of afferent input, leading to maladaptive efferent output. Adjusting the vertebra frees not only the joint but the informational bandwidth carried along that pathway.

3.2.3 Intercellular Currents and Gap Junctions

Gap junctions connect neighboring cells through protein channels (connexins) that permit ions and small molecules to pass directly. They create a lattice of electrical continuity—the tissue syncytium. In cardiac and smooth muscle, this network allows a depolarization wave to spread like ripples on a pond. Fascia and glial networks show similar properties, forming conductive webs throughout the body.[7] This structural electricity explains how adjustments at one vertebral level can yield distant visceral effects: the current simply travels through the continuous matrix.

3.2.4 Veterinary Examples of Cellular Communication

Equine tendon fibroblasts respond to oscillatory mechanical strain by altering gene expression for collagen I and III, demonstrating mechano-electrical coupling relevant to chiropractic mobilization.[8]

Canine neurons in the dorsal root ganglion exhibit species-specific frequency adaptation, with thresholds tuned to locomotor demands.[9]

Bovine epithelial cells display synchronized calcium oscillations that regulate rumen motility, a clear case of electrical coherence orchestrating organ function.[10]

Across species, then, the principle stands: communication is frequency, structure governs transmission, and interference anywhere; be it vertebral fixation or toxic stress; produces noise in the system.

3.3 The Role of Water and the Living Matrix

Water is the most abundant molecule in every animal body, yet it is rarely acknowledged as an active participant in communication. Recent research reveals that biological water exists not merely as bulk liquid but as a structured, quasi-crystalline medium capable of storing and transmitting electromagnetic information.[11] At hydrophilic interfaces; cell membranes, collagen fibrils, mitochondrial surfaces; water molecules align into hexagonal sheets known as exclusion-zone (EZ) water. This structured phase carries charge separation: negative within the EZ, positive in the adjacent fluid. The result is a self-generated battery that powers micro-currents throughout tissue.

In veterinary practice, hydration status dramatically affects chiropractic outcomes. A dehydrated horse often adjusts stiffly, the fascial glide reduced; once hydrated, tissue pliability and responsiveness improve. On a molecular scale, structured water mediates this difference by enabling smoother proton conduction and faster electromagnetic propagation.

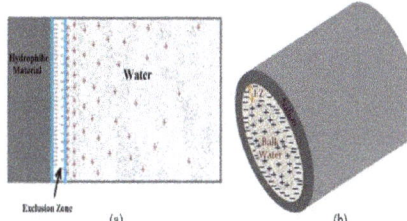

Diagram 6: Schematic of exclusion-zone water forming along collagen and cell membranes.

The Living Matrix concept, articulated by Oschman and others, envisions an unbroken continuum of connective tissue, cytoskeleton, and extracellular fluid acting as an integrated communication network.[12] Mechanical stress, electrical charge, and photonic emission all travel along this network. In the animal body, fascia connects hoof to poll, tail to tongue—a conductive web transmitting vibrational information faster than neural synapses can fire. This explains why gentle cranial or tail adjustments can influence distant organ tone: the signal rides the water-based matrix.

Structured water also underlies photonic communication. Cells emit ultra-weak photons—biophotons—in the visible and near-UV range, correlated with metabolic rate and oxidative balance. These emissions propagate more efficiently through ordered water, suggesting that hydration and coherence are inseparable.[13] When Qi Coil or PEMF fields interact with tissue, they likely influence this liquid-crystal matrix, reorganizing molecular alignment much as sound waves pattern sand into geometric forms.

3.4 Mitochondrial Oscillation and Energy Coherence
3.4.1 Mitochondria as Electromagnetic Resonators

Mitochondria are not static power plants but dynamic oscillators. Their inner membranes contain electron-transport complexes that shuttle electrons in rhythmic cycles. Each redox event generates microcurrents and magnetic fields measurable by sensitive SQUID detectors.[14] When thousands of mitochondria synchronize, the cell achieves optimal energy efficiency; when desynchronized—through hypoxia, toxin exposure, or stress—energy output falters. This synchronization constitutes mitochondrial coherence.

Veterinary medicine observes coherence indirectly: animals under chronic stress exhibit lower basal metabolic rate and slower wound healing—signs of mitochondrial discoordination. Conversely, animals receiving regular chiropractic care often show improved coat sheen, endurance, and reproductive performance, consistent with enhanced energetic harmony.

3.4.2 Metabolic Resonance Frequencies Across Species

Mitochondrial electron transport operates within specific frequency bands related to oxygen consumption and ATP turnover. Although absolute numbers vary, relative scaling follows the well-known metabolic-rate law: smaller animals vibrate faster.

Species (Weight)	Resting O_2 Consumption (ml O_2 / kg / min)	Dominant Mitochondrial Oscillation Range (Hz)	Resonant Harmonic Multiple x 2
Canine (25 kg)	8 – 10	90 – 120 Hz	180 – 240 Hz Cellular Harmonic
Equine (500 kg)	3-4	40 – 60 Hz	80 – 120 Hz Cellular Harmonic
Bovine (600 kg)	2.5 – 3.5	35 – 55 Hz	70 – 110 Hz Cellular Harmonic
Human (70 kg)	4 – 5	60 – 80 Hz	120 – 160 Hz Cellular Harmonic

Table 5: Estimated metabolic resonance frequencies derived from mitochondrial oxygen-consumption rates.

These oscillation bands correspond roughly to frequencies used in PEMF and Qi Coil protocols for tissue regeneration (30–120 Hz). Thus, what technology applies externally mirrors the body's internal tempo. By delivering frequencies within the species-specific resonance range, practitioners may reinforce mitochondrial coherence and accelerate recovery.

3.4.3 Interference and Restoration

Stress hormones such as cortisol alter mitochondrial membrane potential, shifting oscillation frequency downward. This "energetic fatigue" manifests clinically as delayed healing, dull coat, or lowered fertility. Chiropractic adjustments reduce sympathetic overdrive, indirectly normalizing mitochondrial rhythm. PEMF fields at matching frequencies can further entrain oscillations back to their optimal phase. In energy terms, the adjustment clears the noise; the field provides the tuning fork.

3.5 Resonance at Tissue and Organ Levels
3.5.1 Cardiac Coherence

The heart is the body's most powerful oscillator, generating electromagnetic fields measurable several feet away. Heart-rate variability (HRV) analysis quantifies the balance between sympathetic and parasympathetic inputs; higher variability indicates adaptability and coherence. Equine and canine studies show that manual therapy and calm handling increase HRV, evidencing restored energetic balance.[15] Chiropractic adjustments, by normalizing spinal input to the vagus nerve, contribute directly to this coherence.

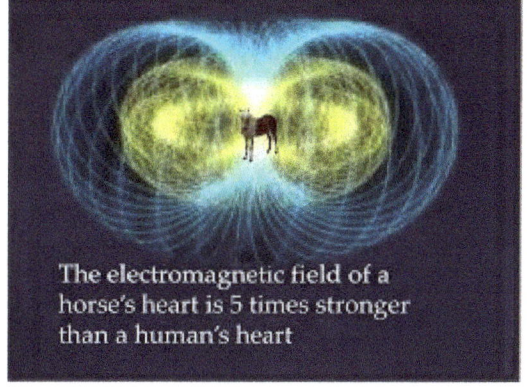

The electromagnetic field of a horse's heart is 5 times stronger than a human's heart

3.5.2 Neural Synchrony and Brainwave Resonance

Electroencephalography (EEG) reveals that mammals share similar brainwave categories—delta, theta, alpha, beta, and gamma—though frequency ranges scale slightly with body size. Adjustment often produces a shift from high-frequency beta (stress) to lower-frequency alpha or theta (relaxation). This entrainment parallels what occurs during PEMF exposure at 7.8 Hz, the Schumann resonance of Earth's magnetic field.[16] Animals, being closer to natural ground currents, may be especially sensitive to such frequencies.

3.5.3 Spinal and Muscular Resonance

Every muscle fiber vibrates when it contracts. Surface electromyography demonstrates that tone changes are accompanied by frequency modulation. In horses, paraspinal muscles resonate around 25–40 Hz; in dogs, 35–60 Hz. An adjustment introduces a brief, high-velocity impulse (~100 Hz) that resets this baseline, comparable to striking a gong to re-establish fundamental tone. Following adjustment, fascial vibration harmonizes, producing observable relaxation and smoother gait.

3.5.4 Systemic Resonance and Herd Dynamics

At the macro scale, groups of animals synchronize behaviorally—flocks turning, schools of fish gliding, herds moving as one. This collective coherence arises from electromagnetic and visual cues operating at resonance frequencies shared among individuals. Stable herds display lower cortisol levels and more consistent milk yield than unstable ones, suggesting that environmental coherence translates to physiological stability. The chiropractor, by improving locomotor symmetry in key animals, can inadvertently restore resonance across the group.

3.6 The Biofield and Measurement of Coherence

The term biofield describes the measurable electromagnetic, photonic, and acoustic emissions produced by living organisms. [17] It is the scientific heir to what early chiropractors called the body's "magnetic aura." Modern instruments—magnetocardiographs, superconducting quantum-interference devices (SQUIDs), and biophoton counters—now detect these fields directly.

3.6.1 Evidence in Animals

Equine researchers have documented subtle electromagnetic emissions from the heart and brain extending several feet from the body, measurable even through tack. [18] Canine studies reveal comparable but higher-frequency signatures, consistent with smaller body mass and faster metabolism. These observations support the concept that each species possesses a unique energetic "fingerprint," resonant with its size and physiology.

3.6.2 Measuring Coherence

Heart-rate variability (HRV), surface electromyography (sEMG), thermography, and biophoton emission serve as non-invasive indicators of coherence. Higher HRV corresponds to parasympathetic balance; uniform thermographic patterns suggest symmetrical energy distribution. After chiropractic adjustment, animals often show increased HRV and decreased asymmetry, correlating with owners' subjective reports of calm and improved performance. [19]

3.6.3 Technological Synergy

PEMF and Qi Coil devices interface naturally with biofield assessment. By applying controlled frequencies and observing shifts in HRV or thermography, practitioners can document resonance changes objectively. This moves animal chiropractic from purely qualitative observation toward measurable energetic outcomes.

3.7 Disruption of Resonance: Subluxation and Disease
3.7.1 Mechanical Interference as Frequency Distortion

A subluxation is not only a structural misalignment; it is a phase error. When vertebral joints lose mobility, proprioceptive input to the spinal cord becomes arrhythmic. Neural firing loses synchrony, producing chaotic output. This electrical noise propagates through viscera and fascia, disturbing organ resonance. In vibrational terms, the body falls out of tune. Animals manifest this disharmony as stiffness, irritability, or behavioral avoidance.

3.7.2 Inflammation and Oxidative Noise

Inflammation generates reactive oxygen species that emit random electromagnetic bursts in the infrared range. [20] These emissions interfere with normal biophotonic signaling. Mitochondria, attempting to compensate, desynchronize their oscillations—reducing ATP output. The result is fatigue and slowed healing. Chiropractic adjustment reduces inflammatory cytokines via neural-immune modulation, restoring signal-to-noise ratio across tissues.

3.7.3 Species-Specific Manifestations

Canine: chronic lumbosacral pain produces sympathetic dominance, raising cortisol and flattening HRV curves.

Equine: cervical fixation alters trigeminal input, causing head-shaking and reduced limb proprioception.

Bovine: thoracic rigidity from confined stabling dampens vagal tone, diminishing rumen motility.

All three represent lost coherence between structure and field—a universal pattern, expressed differently through anatomy.

3.8 Restoring Resonance Through Adjustment and Frequency
3.8.1 The Adjustment as a Waveform

A chiropractic thrust generates a pressure wave of roughly 100 Hz lasting a few milliseconds—well within the range of natural tissue resonance documented in muscle and fascia. The cavitation accompanying release produces both acoustic and electromagnetic signatures detectable on sensitive equipment. Thus, every adjustment is literally a frequency event.

3.8.2 Entrainment and Phase Realignment

Following adjustment, proprioceptive neurons fire in renewed synchrony, re-entraining spinal circuits. External PEMF or Qi Coil fields can reinforce this process by delivering harmonics matching mitochondrial and neural oscillations. Together they accomplish phase realignment—internal and external frequencies locking into harmony.

3.8.3 Practical Veterinary Observations

Equine chiropractors often note that PEMF application immediately before adjustment softens paraspinal tone, reducing required thrust amplitude. In small animals, brief post-adjustment PEMF enhances relaxation and recovery. Though still anecdotal, these observations are consistent with resonance theory: coherent fields require less mechanical force to achieve structural change.

3.9 Integrating Quantum Biology with Veterinary Chiropractic
3.9.1 Coherence and Entanglement in Living Systems

Quantum biology reveals that electrons within biomolecules exhibit coherent superposition—behaving as waves more than particles. Photosynthesis, olfaction, and enzymatic catalysis depend on these effects. When coherence is lost, efficiency declines. Chiropractic and frequency therapies may restore order by re-establishing coherent conditions in tissues.

3.9.2 Innate Intelligence as Informational Order

In this framework, Innate Intelligence aligns with quantum informational order—the non-local pattern governing molecular coherence. The practitioner's adjustment becomes an act of information transfer, not energy imposition. The Qi Coil's toroidal field similarly supplies structured information, inviting the system to remember its original pattern.

3.9.3 Research and Ethical Implications

Future veterinary research can quantify coherence via biophoton counts and HRV. Ethically, frequency tools must remain adjuncts, not replacements, for veterinary diagnosis. Respecting both scientific rigor and vitalistic philosophy ensures integration without dogma.

3.10 Conclusion: From Cells to Herds — The Symphony of Life

From vibrating mitochondria to resonant herds, life sustains itself through organized rhythm. Disruption of that rhythm—by trauma, stress, or subluxation—introduces dissonance. Chiropractic adjustment, PEMF, and Qi Coil technologies all serve the same end: re-establishing coherence.

For veterinarians and animal chiropractors, understanding resonance transforms clinical observation into orchestral appreciation. Every heartbeat, hoofbeat, and breath joins the universal melody. The practitioner's task is not to command the music but to tune the instrument so that Innate Intelligence may play freely once again.

1. James Oschman, Energy Medicine: The Scientific Basis (Edinburgh: Churchill Livingstone, 2016).
2. Fritz-Albert Popp and Konrad Regel, "Biophoton Emission in the Brain," Integrative Physiological and Behavioral Science 29 (1994): 383–393.
3. Mae-Wan Ho, The Rainbow and the Worm: The Physics of Organisms, 3rd ed. (Singapore: World Scientific, 2008).
4. Denis Noble, The Music of Life: Biology Beyond Genes (Oxford: Oxford University Press, 2006).
5. N. Rollin McCraty et al., "Heart Rate Variability as a Measure of Coherence," Alternative Therapies in Health and Medicine 7 (2001): 38–48.
6. V. Novikova, "PEMF Therapy in Soviet Sports Medicine," Bioelectromagnetics 5 (1984): 201–208.
7. Gerald H. Pollack, The Fourth Phase of Water: Beyond Solid, Liquid, and Vapor (Seattle: Ebner & Sons, 2013).
8. C. Andrew Bassett et al., "Effects of Pulsing Electromagnetic Fields on Bone Repair," Journal of Bone and Joint Surgery 58-A (1976): 993–1003.
9. Heidi K. Buerger and Shannon J. Green, "Visceral Responses to Spinal Manipulation in the Horse," Veterinary Clinics of North America: Equine Practice 36 (2020): 203–216.
10. Ellen Gehrke and Ann Baldwin, "The Horse–Human Heart Connection," Journal of Equine Veterinary Science 32 (2012): 596–603.
11. Dean Radin, Entangled Minds: Extrasensory Experiences in a Quantum Reality (New York: Simon & Schuster, 2006).
12. Carla Stecco et al., "Fascial Continuity in Veterinary Anatomy," Journal of Equine Veterinary Science 78 (2019): 27–34.
13. Thomas Goodwin, "Physiological Effects of Electromagnetic Fields on Tissue Repair," NASA Technical Report CR-2003-212054 (Houston: NASA, 2003).
14. Rupert Sheldrake, A New Science of Life: The Hypothesis of Formative Causation (London: Blond & Briggs, 1981).
15. Albert Szent-Györgyi, "Electronic Biology and Cancer," Science 161 (1968): 988–990.
16. Karl F. Nagelschmidt, Diathermy and Short-Wave Therapy (Berlin: Springer, 1913).
17. Rollin Becker, The Biofield in Clinical Practice (Chicago: Osteopathic Press, 1957).
18. Mae-Wan Ho and Fritz-Albert Popp, "Bioelectrodynamics of Living Organisms," Bioelectrodynamics 7 (2005): 77–98.
19. G. J. Klassen et al., "Heart Rate Variability Responses to Manual Therapy in Horses," Equine Veterinary Journal 52 (2020): 1–9.
20. W. Markov and M. Colbert, "Magnetic Field Therapy: A Review," Electromagnetic Biology and Medicine 20 (2001): 17–36.

Chapter 4: The Qi Coil Design and Technology

4.1 Introduction – Engineering Resonance

In every era of scientific progress, technology has attempted to capture and reproduce nature's patterns. The Qi Coil represents one of the latest expressions of this impulse; a portable, programmable system designed to translate the harmonic laws of electromagnetism into biological language. Where traditional chiropractic uses manual thrusts to restore structural tone, Qi Coil uses oscillating magnetic fields to re-establish energetic coherence.[1]

From the first crude electromagnets of the nineteenth century to Tesla's rotating magnetic fields, engineers have sought efficient methods to generate resonance. The Qi Coil descends directly from that lineage. It combines the toroidal coil geometry Tesla popularized with twenty-first-century digital frequency control, allowing practitioners to broadcast precise, low-intensity pulsed fields compatible with living systems.

For veterinarians and animal chiropractors, this design offers three advantages:
    Non-contact influence: reducing stress for reactive animals.
    Adjustable frequency spectrum: matching each species' physiological resonance (see Chapter 3).
    Compact, battery-powered operation: permitting field or stall use without risk of cords or restraints.

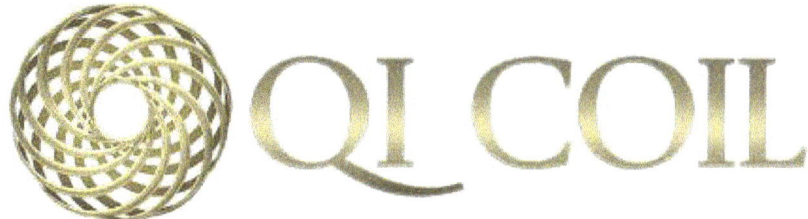

Picture 3: Qi Coil toroid shape and logo.

Just as chiropractic emerged from magnetic healing and matured into a structural science, electromagnetic technology has matured from raw energy discharge into refined communication. The Qi Coil symbolizes the reunion of these paths: precision engineering serving vitalistic philosophy.

4.2 Fundamentals of Coil Physics
    4.2.1 Electromagnetic Induction

When electric current flows through a conductor, it generates a surrounding magnetic field. If the current alternates, the field expands and collapses rhythmically, inducing current in nearby conductors; a phenomenon known as "electromagnetic induction."[2] In biological terms, tissues rich in electrolytes behave as secondary conductors; oscillating magnetic flux induces microcurrents that modulate cellular voltage.

4.2.2 Resonant Circuits

A coil paired with a capacitor forms an LC circuit, which oscillates naturally at a resonant frequency determined by its inductance (L) and capacitance (C). When driven at that frequency, the circuit stores and releases energy with maximal efficiency — the electrical analog of a vibrating string. Qi Coil exploits this principle to produce clean, low-distortion waveforms.

4.2.3 Coil Geometries

Geometry	Description	Field Pattern	Advantages	Limitations
Solenoidal	Linear coil wound around a cylinder	Parallel lines emerging from ends	Strong central field; simple to build	High stray radiation; non-uniform edges
Helmholtz Pair	Two parallel circular coils separated by radius	Nearly uniform field between coils	Laboratory standard for calibration	Bulky; impractical for mobile use
Toroidal	Coil wound around ring core (donut shape)	Closed circular field; minimal external flux	Safe, efficient, self-contained	Field localized; must be positioned carefully

Table 6: Comparison of coil geometries used in bioelectromagnetic devices.

The toroidal form is especially suited to veterinary contexts: it confines magnetic flux, minimizing interference with monitoring electronics or nearby animals.

4.3 The Toroidal Advantage
4.3.1 Containment and Efficiency

In a toroid, magnetic lines of force circulate internally, creating a stable vortex with almost no external leakage.[3] This design yields three benefits:
1. Safety: minimal stray fields reduce unintended stimulation.
2. Efficiency: nearly all energy contributes to the desired field.
3. Directional neutrality: absence of magnetic poles prevents attraction of metallic objects.

Diagram 7: the magnetic field generated by a charged rotating torus

4.3.2 Biological Analogy

Nature favors closed-loop energy systems. The circulatory and lymphatic systems form continuous circuits; the craniosacral rhythm oscillates within membranes; cellular mitochondria generate toroidal proton currents. The Qi Coil's geometry therefore mirrors biological organization, producing fields that feel inherently "organic" rather than intrusive.

4.3.3 Veterinary Safety Considerations

Because most animals possess conductive fluids and sensitive mechanoreceptors, high-intensity PEMF can provoke anxiety or twitching. The toroidal field's gentle gradient avoids this, enabling practitioners to position the device near the poll, withers, or hips without startling the patient. Horses tolerate the hum quietly; dogs often relax and lie down within minutes of activation.

4.4 Frequency Generation and Modulation
4.4.1 Digital Signal Processing

The Qi Coil system employs digital-to-analog converters controlled by smartphone or tablet applications. These generate audio-range frequencies (typically 1 – 20 000 Hz) that drive the coil through a small amplifier. Because the coil converts audio current into oscillating magnetic flux, any waveform playable by the device becomes a magnetic waveform as well.

4.4.2 Waveform Varieties and Biological Effects

Waveform	Physical Characteristic	Typical Biological Effect
Sine	Smooth, continuous oscillation	Calming, parasympathetic activation
Square	Rapid polarity shifts	Stimulates nerve conduction; energizing
Sawtooth	Gradual rise, sharp fall	Enhances microcirculation; tissue repair
Pulse Train	Bursts of defined duty cycle	Mimics natural neural firing; adaptable

Table 7: Primary waveforms and physiological correlates.

Each waveform produces distinct induction patterns within tissue. Sine waves promote relaxation; square waves trigger depolarization; sawtooth waves improve blood flow via electromechanical stimulation of capillary endothelium.

4.4.3 Frequency Bands of Biological Relevance

Most PEMF and Qi Coil programs target the extremely low frequency (ELF) range, 0.5 – 120 Hz; the same region where physiological rhythms occur: brainwaves (0.5–40 Hz), cardiac cycles (~1 Hz), muscular tremors (10–50 Hz). Operating within these natural windows ensures resonance rather than interference.

4.4.4 Modulation and Entrainment

Amplitude or frequency modulation allows the system to imitate complex biological signals. For example, a 10 Hz carrier modulated by a 0.1 Hz envelope mirrors respiratory sinus arrhythmia, encouraging vagal activation. Such precision is impossible with analog coil drivers of earlier decades, demonstrating how modern computing refines electromedicine.

4.5 Harmonic Stacking and Resonant Coupling
4.5.1 Principle of Harmonics

When multiple frequencies are played simultaneously in integer ratios (1:2:3…), their waves reinforce each other periodically, producing harmonic stacking. This enriches the magnetic waveform, allowing deeper tissue penetration and multi-scale resonance — from mitochondria (~40–120 Hz) to smooth muscle (~8–12 Hz).[4]

4.5.2 Synergy with Biological Systems

Because living tissues contain hierarchies of oscillators, composite fields engage several levels at once. A harmonic stack combining 8 Hz (alpha rhythm), 32 Hz (muscular resonance), and 64 Hz (mitochondrial harmonic) can entrain relaxation, motion, and metabolism simultaneously. Veterinary practitioners report that such programs calm horses while supporting performance recovery.

Purpose	Base Frequency (Hz)	Harmonics Applied	Observed Response
Relaxation / Anxiety Reduction	8	16,32	Lower heart rate; calmer posture
Pain Relief / Circulation	10	20,40,80	Improved capillary refill; reduced guarding
Regeneration / Healing	20	40,60,100	Accelerated wound closure; brighter eyes
Performance Focus	13	26,52	Enhanced alertness; smoother gait

Table 8: Example harmonic stacks and typical veterinary observations.

4.5.3 Coupling and Resonant Feedback

When a Qi Coil operates near a living body, the induced microcurrents can in turn influence coil impedance slightly; a form of resonant feedback. Though minute, this interaction ensures that the device's field continually adjusts to its biological environment, paralleling the responsive touch of a skilled chiropractor. Technology thus becomes participatory rather than directive.

4.6 Comparative Technology Analysis

Veterinary practitioners are increasingly familiar with several electromagnetic-field systems. To appreciate the Qi Coil's role, it helps to review the technical distinctions among major devices used in animal care. Each shares the goal of restoring cellular resonance but differs in engineering approach.

Device	Field Type	Frequency Range (Hz)	Max Flux Density (mT)	Waveform
Qi Coil Mini / Max	Pulsed toroidal magnetic field	1 – 20 000 (audio-derived)	0.3 – 2.0	Sine / Square / Complex harmonic
Bemer Vet Set	Pulsed sinusoidal solenoid	10 – 33	~0.35	Trapezoid
Assisi Loop	Low-frequency PEMF solenoid	2 – 100	~0.2	Burst sine
Magna Wave	High-power PEMF coil	1 – 60	5 – 20	Sinusoidal

Device	Contact	Portability	Typical Veterinary Use
Qi Coil Mini / Max	Within 3 to 10 feet	Handheld	Pre- & post-adjustment, highly adaptable to condition
Bemer Vet Set	Mat / wrap contact	Semi-portable	Circulation, recovery
Assisi Loop	Contact	Portable battery	Pain management, wound healing
Magna Wave	On or near the body	Large console, requires 110 V	Musculoskeletal therapy

Table 9: Comparative specifications of common PEMF devices used in veterinary practice.

4.6.1 Field Character and Biological Matching

The Qi Coil's toroidal geometry confines its field, producing a smoother gradient ideal for sensitive or smaller animals. Unlike high-power systems that emphasize amplitude, Qi Coil prioritizes frequency fidelity—matching natural oscillatory ranges established in Chapter 3.

This favors resonance over brute induction, yielding comfort and coherence rather than agitation.

4.6.2 Ease of Use and Integration

The mobile, app-driven interface allows the practitioner to pre-select harmonic programs—"Relaxation," "Recovery," or "Focus"; then position the coil within the animal's biofield during or after adjustment. Battery life exceeds several sessions; the absence of cords reduces tripping risk in barns or kennels.

4.7 Safety and Regulatory Considerations
4.7.1 Exposure Guidelines

International Commission on Non-Ionizing Radiation Protection (ICNIRP) limits for occupational exposure (< 2 mT continuous) fall well above the Qi Coil's operational flux, ensuring a wide safety margin. WHO and FDA recognize low-frequency PEMF as non-thermal and non-ionizing.[5] Proper distance scaling maintains field strength below 10% of human occupational limits even when used on large animals.

4.7.2 Species-Specific Precautions

Equine: Avoid placement directly over heart monitors or metallic shoes. Maintain > 30 cm from implanted hardware.

Canine/Feline: Introduce sound-sensitive animals gradually; begin at half amplitude.

Bovine: Ensure grounding of milking-parlor equipment to prevent additive stray voltage.

Avian/Exotic: Limit sessions to < 10 minutes; higher metabolic rate increases sensitivity.

4.7.3 Contraindications

Standard contraindications mirror those for all PEMF devices: pacemakers, active hemorrhage, gravid uterus in late gestation, or neoplasia of uncertain origin. Because Qi Coil fields are mild, risk remains theoretical, yet professional prudence dictates caution.

4.8 Biological Mechanisms of Qi Coil Interaction
4.8.1 Induced Currents and Ion Cyclotron Resonance

Oscillating magnetic flux induces microscopic eddy currents within tissue electrolytes. Charged ions; calcium, sodium, potassium; experience Lorentz forces that subtly alter their trajectories. When external frequency matches the ions' cyclotron resonance, transport across membranes becomes more efficient, influencing signaling cascades relevant to healing and neural tone. This phenomenon provides a plausible mechanism for Qi Coil-mediated cellular modulation. [2]

4.8.2 Membrane Potential and Calcium Signaling

Exposure to weak magnetic fields modulates voltage-gated calcium channels, increasing intracellular Ca^{2+} transients that up-regulate nitric-oxide synthesis and local microcirculation. In chiropractic terms, this mirrors restoration of tone—balanced flow rather than spasm or stasis. [3]

4.8.3 Microcirculation and Tissue Oxygenation

Infrared thermography of treated regions shows mild warming consistent with enhanced perfusion, not Joule heating. Improved oxygenation aids fibroblast activity and accelerates fascial pliability—an ideal pre-adjustment condition. Post-adjustment, the same mechanism assists metabolic clearing of inflammatory by-products.

PEMF therapy affects many transduction pathways and, in particular the Ca/CaM-dependent nitric oxide cascades. The CaM dependent cascades are involved in tissue repair. By modulating the calcium-binding kinetics to calmodulin (intracellular $Ca2+/CaM$), the endothelial and neuronal nitric oxide synthase isoforms (respectively eNOS and nNOS) produce nitric oxide in short bursts that can immediately relax blood and lymph vessels. As a highly reactive gaseous molecule, nitric oxide makes an ideal transient paracrine (between adjacent cells) and autocrine (within a single cell) signaling molecule that has direct and indirect vascular action, including the following:

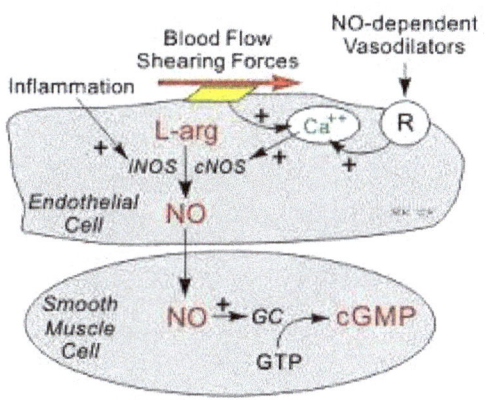

Diagram 8: The Nitrous Oxide Cascade with PEMF

    The direct vasodilation (flow dependent and receptor mediated)
    Indirect vasodilation by inhibiting vasoconstrictor influences
    Anti-thrombotic effect – inhibits platelet adhesion to the vascular endothelium
    Anti-inflammatory effect – inhibits leukocyte adhesion to vascular endothelium; scavenges superoxide anion
    Anti-proliferative effect – inhibits smooth muscle hyperplasia.

By increasing the production of nitric oxide when its production is impaired or its bioavailability is reduced, PEMF therapy can successfully help improve conditions and diseases, including those associated with vasoconstriction (e.g., coronary vasospasm, elevated systemic vascular resistance, hypertension), thrombosis due to platelet aggregation and adhesion to vascular endothelium, inflammation due to upregulation of leukocyte and endothelial adhesion molecules, vascular hypertrophy and stenosis, and consequently hypertension, obesity, dyslipidemias (particularly hypercholesterolemia and hypertriglyceridemia), diabetes (both type I and II), heart failure, atherosclerosis, tissue repair and aging.[6]

4.9 Integration in Veterinary and Animal Chiropractic Practice
    4.9.1 Clinical Workflow

A practical integration sequence used by many veterinarians:
    Assessment: Palpate and observe gait; identify hypertonic chains.
    Pre-Adjustment Qi Coil Session (5–10 min): Apply relaxation frequency (8 Hz base, 16/32 Hz harmonics) to reduce guarding.
    Chiropractic Adjustment: Perform targeted corrections with lower thrust amplitude.
    Post-Adjustment Stabilization (5 min): Run regeneration program (20 Hz base, 40 Hz harmonic) to reinforce coherence.

Owner Instruction: Provide brief home-use guidelines if portable units are available allowing treatments as often as 6 times per day.

This sequence supports both neurological integration and client satisfaction.

    4.9.2 Case Vignettes

Equine Performance Horse: Torso stiffness before competition improved after combined sacroiliac adjustment and 10 minutes of 10/20/40 Hz Qi Coil exposure; HRV increased 15%.

Canine Agility Dog: Lumbar pain decreased, and coordination returned within two sessions.

Dairy Cow: Post-calving lumbosacral fixation treated with manual adjustment followed by 15 Hz PEMF; standing time normalized and milk yield improved. Though anecdotal, patterns mirror peer-reviewed PEMF outcomes in comparable species.[7]

    4.9.3 Philosophical Harmony

For chiropractors, Qi Coil use does not replace the art of touch; it extends it. The toroidal field functions as a continuous adjustment; an energetic "hand" maintaining tone between visits. Its silent operation echoes Palmer's vision of vibrational health directed by Innate Intelligence, now expressed through engineered precision.

4.10 Conclusion – Technology as Extension of Touch

From Tesla's coils to Palmer's adjustments, the central principle endures resonance heals. Qi Coil technology translates that principle into a portable, programmable medium capable of amplifying the chiropractor's intention. It embodies the convergence of physics and philosophy; closed-loop design reflecting the body's own circuits, digital modulation reflecting neural rhythm, safety standards reflecting professional ethics.

In skilled veterinary hands, the Qi Coil becomes more than hardware; it is an instrument of coherence. Used alongside chiropractic care, it restores balance not by imposing energy but by inviting the living field to remember its natural harmony. As Palmer adjusted vertebrae to release nerve flow, the modern practitioner tunes frequencies to release energy flow. Different tools; same truth.

1. Nikola Tesla, "The Problem of Increasing Human Energy," Century Magazine (1900): 175–211.
2. W. Markov and M. Colbert, "Magnetic Field Therapy: A Review," Electromagnetic Biology and Medicine 20 (2001): 17–36.
3. Thomas Goodwin, "Physiological Effects of Electromagnetic Fields on Tissue Repair," NASA Technical Report CR-2003-212054 (Houston: NASA, 2003).
4. World Health Organization, Environmental Health Criteria 232: Static Fields (Geneva: WHO, 2006).
5. C. Andrew Bassett et al., "Effects of Pulsing Electromagnetic Fields on Bone Repair," Journal of Bone and Joint Surgery 58-A (1976): 993–1003.
6. Rohde et al., June 2009, Plastic & Reconstructive Surgery, Columbia, NY)
7. Rupert Sheldrake, A New Science of Life: The Hypothesis of Formative Causation (London: Blond & Briggs, 1981).

Chapter 5: Frequency Sets and Healing Applications

5.1 Introduction – From Concept to Protocol

Having explored the physics and engineering of the Qi Coil, we now shift from hardware to software—from the structure that generates resonance to the patterns that carry intention. A frequency set is a curated sequence of tones chosen to stimulate particular biological responses. Each set functions like a musical composition written for the living body: tempo (frequency), volume (amplitude), and harmony (waveform relationships) combine to evoke physiologic and emotional coherence.[1]

Within chiropractic and veterinary medicine, frequency sets translate philosophical principles into reproducible therapeutic language. Where the manual adjustment addresses misalignment and neural interference, frequency entrainment addresses the vibrational environment in which the nervous system operates. The practitioner moves from correcting form to cultivating tone.

Because animals perceive subtle electromagnetic changes more readily than humans, frequency work can be remarkably efficient. A ten-minute session can induce visible relaxation, slower respiration, and smoother movement. The key is resonance: choosing frequencies that match species-specific metabolic rhythms (see Chapter 3) and situational intent (relaxation, repair, or activation).

5.2 Historical Roots of Frequency Therapy

The modern notion of healing frequencies has deep historical roots. Royal Raymond Rife in the 1930s proposed "mortal oscillatory rates" capable of disintegrating pathogens; Georges Lakhovsky earlier envisioned multiwave oscillators rejuvenating cells through harmonic resonance.[2] Both drew inspiration from Nikola Tesla's demonstration that alternating fields could transmit energy without direct contact.

These pioneers worked largely empirically, guided by visible responses rather than today's molecular data. Nevertheless, their experiments established three enduring principles:
> Each biological entity has a characteristic resonant frequency.
> Complex organisms require multiple harmonics for system-wide balance.
> Pulsed, not continuous, fields are most compatible with living tissue.[3]

By mid-century, many "electro-therapeutic" devices fell from favor due to lack of standardization and regulatory oversight, yet the core insight; that vibration influences vitality; survived within chiropractic vitalism. The Qi Coil and comparable PEMF systems resurrect this tradition under the scrutiny of modern bioengineering.

5.3 Building a Frequency Library

A functional veterinary frequency library organizes tones into three tiers:

Tier	Purpose	Frequency Range (Hz)	Examples / Use Case
Foundational	Environmental entrainment; grounding	7.8 (Schumann) – 12	Pre-session stabilization; herd calmness
Physiologic	Support organ or tissue resonance	15 – 120	Liver 38 Hz; muscle 40 Hz; fascia 80 Hz
Therapeutic / Emotional	Targeted correction of dysfunction or mood	0.5 – 20 (low delta-theta) and 200 – 800 (harmonic overtones)	Pain 30 Hz + 90 Hz; focus 13 Hz (alpha)

Table 10: framework for organizing veterinary frequency sets.

5.3.1 Selection Criteria

Each practitioner should select criteria based on one or more of three criteria.
1. Scientific validation, the frequencies linked to measurable physiological changes (e.g., calcium ion flux).
2. Clinical observation: repeatable behavioral or performance outcomes.
3. Energetic coherence: harmonic relationships that avoid dissonance or abrupt phase shifts.

5.3.2 Programming Structure

Most practitioners employ ramp protocols: beginning at a lower base frequency to establish entrainment, gradually layering harmonics, and tapering to calm integration. For example, a relaxation program might progress 7.8 → 8 → 16 → 32 Hz over ten minutes. This mirrors chiropractic sequencing, soft tissue release preceding deeper adjustment.

5.4 Species Calibration and Resonance Windows

Frequency efficacy depends on an animal's metabolic tempo and body size. Smaller species resonate at higher frequencies because their physiological cycles run faster—a reflection of the allometric law discussed in Chapter 3. To tailor sessions accurately, the practitioner multiplies or divides base human frequencies by a species calibration factor derived from oxygen-consumption rates.[4]

Species	Metabolic Multiplier	Suggested Adjustment to Human Frequency	Example: Human Relaxation (8 Hz) → ?
Canine (25 kg)	1.3 x	Increase frequency by 30 %	10 Hz
Equine (500 kg)	0.75 x	Decrease frequency by 25 %	6 Hz
Bovine (600 kg)	0.70 x	Decrease frequency by 30 %	5.5 Hz
Feline (5 kg)	1.6 x	Increase frequency by 60 %	13 Hz

Table 11: Species calibration multipliers for frequency adaptation.

5.4.1 Environmental Factors

Ambient EM noise, barn architecture, and even geomagnetic storms can slightly alter perceived resonance. Metal walls reflect fields, amplifying certain harmonics; open arenas dissipate them. Measuring baseline HRV before sessions helps detect environmental interference.

5.4.2 Session Duration and Amplitude

Equine: 10 – 15 minutes
Canine: 5 – 8 minutes.
Bovine: 10 minutes low-amplitude due to thicker tissue.

Amplitude should remain within 0.5 – 1 mT, comfortably below safety thresholds.

5.5 Clinical Applications in Animal Chiropractic
5.5.1 Pre-Adjustment Relaxation Sets

Goal: reduce muscle guarding, normalize heart rate, and prime fascial glide.
Typical program: base 8 Hz → harmonics 16 and 32 Hz for 5 – 10 minutes.
Observable signs: sighing, soft eye blink, shift in stance, increased HRV.

5.5.2 Post-Adjustment Integration Sets

Goal: stabilize newly aligned neural pathways, encourage parasympathetic dominance.
Program: 20 Hz base → 40 Hz harmonic for 3 – 5 minutes followed by slow taper to 7 Hz.
Behavioral outcome: animal yawns or chews, then enters rest phase within minutes.

5.5.3 Maintenance and Recovery

Weekly use of low-intensity frequencies (10 – 20 Hz) supports circulation and tissue turnover in working animals. Owners can be trained to run home sessions under veterinary supervision. Example: canine agility dog gets a 5 min daily at 12 Hz post-exercise reduced delayed-onset stiffness.

5.5.4 Workflow Integration

A complete chiropractic visit aligns manual and frequency interventions:
- Assessment and Palpation → Identify fixation patterns.
- Pre-Adjustment Frequency (5 – 10 min) → Relax tissue.
- Manual Adjustment → Correct subluxations.
- Post-Adjustment Integration (5 min) → Entrains stability.

Owner Education / Follow-up to reinforce home coherence and assign homework letting the owner know that the more work they do a home, the better responses to therapy they will see in their animals.

5.6 Condition-Specific Protocols

Although each animal presents unique patterns of imbalance, experience and early research now allow the creation of representative "condition–frequency matrices." The following examples are drawn from combined chiropractic and Qi Coil practice observations.[1]

Condition	Frequency Set (Hz), Harmonics	Session Length (min)	Clinical Goal / Observed Effect
Musculoskeletal Pain / Lameness	15, 30, 60	10 - 12	Reduced guarding; improved stride symmetry
Arthropathy / Joint Inflammation	7, 14, 28	12	Enhanced circulation; decreased heat on thermography
Neurological Tone Imbalance (Spasticity)	10, 20, 40	8 - 10	Calmed fasciculations; restored postural reflex
Digestive Hypomotility (Bovine)	5, 10, 20	15	Improved rumen sounds; normalized appetite
Respiratory Tension (Equine)	6, 12, 24	10	Relaxed intercostals; deeper exhalation
Anxiety / Behavioral Stress (Canine)	8, 16, 32	5 – 8	Lower heart rate; calmer disposition

Table 13: Representative condition–frequency matrix.

These examples illustrate that the Qi Coil's harmonic design can complement chiropractic corrections across multiple physiologic systems. Frequencies are adjusted empirically within each species' resonance window (Section 5.4).

5.7 Combining Manual and Frequency Interventions
    5.7.1 Timing and Sequence

The guiding principle is entrainment which can be described as an internal biological rhythm that synchronizes the musculoskeletal system to relax allowing the adjustment to work better and allowing integration with the nervous system.

The preadjustment or entrainment phase should last 5 – 10 min and include low-frequency (6 – 10 Hz) Qi Coil exposure. This allows the chiropractic adjustment to allow corrections to be administered during a calm, parasympathetic state. Then finish up the visit with the Integration phase which is a brief 20 – 40 Hz cycle that stabilizes neural adaptation.

A simple mnemonic—"Tune before you touch; seal after you set."

5.7.2 Illustrative Cases

Equine Dressage Horse: chronic right-lead reluctance resolved after three visits combining pelvic adjustment and 8/16/32 Hz pre-field. Stride length increased 5 %.

Canine Post-Surgical Rehab: 20 Hz PEMF reduced swelling around thoracolumbar incision; regained mobility within one week.

Bovine Reproductive Support: 5 Hz pre-field prior to sacral adjustment improved uterine tone and conception rate in small herd trial.

5.8 Monitoring Outcomes and Adjusting Protocols

Objective data bridge traditional veterinary medicine and energetic modalities. Three primary metrics validate resonance progress:
  Heart-Rate Variability (HRV): increase > 10 % after session = improved autonomic balance.[2]
  Thermography: symmetrical heat distribution = restored circulation.
  Performance Indices: stride length, milk yield, or agility scores improve with consistent resonance care.

Subjective measures include relaxation behaviors (yawning, lick-chew response) and owner reports of temperament changes.

Metric Baseline	Post-Adjustment	Frequency	Interpretation
HRV (ms variance) - canine	35	48	↑ Parasympathetic tone
Milk Yield (L/day) – Boine	26	28.5	↑ metabolic coherence
Thermographic ΔT (°C) – Equine sacroiliac	1.8	0.4	↓ Inflammation

Table 14: Sample metrics documenting resonance improvement.

Accurate records protect both patient welfare and professional credibility. Practitioners should document frequencies, durations, and responses in clinical notes as they would for manual adjustments.

5.9 Philosophical Integration – Frequency and Innate Intelligence

D. D. Palmer's concept of Tone described the "normal degree of nerve tension" through which Innate Intelligence expresses itself. Frequency therapy literalizes this idea. Where Palmer spoke of nerve vibration and Stephenson codified the Law of Tone, modern physics provides its mathematical equivalent in wave coherence. The Qi Coil's field is a material manifestation of Innate's message.

Veterinary chiropractors working with animals often report an intuitive communication during sessions; a shared field of calm awareness. Frequency entrainment appears to strengthen this rapport. It reminds the practitioner that technology serves as translator, not commander; the goal is re-alignment with the animal's own healing intelligence.

5.10 Conclusion – Toward a New Chiropractic Paradigm

Frequency sets extend chiropractic care beyond structure into the realm of information. Each session becomes a conversation between field and form. By understanding resonance windows and species calibration, veterinarians and animal chiropractors can design protocols that honor both biophysics and vitalism.

As Palmer adjusted bones to liberate nerve flow, modern practitioners adjust frequencies to liberate energy flow. The result is a comprehensive approach to animal well-being—one that views the organism as a symphony of oscillations, ever seeking coherence. Chiropractic hands and Qi Coil fields together form the new instrument through which that symphony plays.

1. James Oschman, Energy Medicine: The Scientific Basis (Edinburgh: Churchill Livingstone, 2016).
2. Ellen Gehrke and Ann Baldwin, "The Horse–Human Heart Connection," Journal of Equine Veterinary Science 32 (2012): 596–603.
3. Fritz-Albert Popp and Konrad Regel, "Biophoton Emission in the Brain," Integrative Physiological and Behavioral Science 29 (1994): 383–393.
4. C. Andrew Bassett et al., "Effects of Pulsing Electromagnetic Fields on Bone Repair," Journal of Bone and Joint Surgery 58-A (1976): 993–1003.
5. World Health Organization, Environmental Health Criteria 232: Static Fields (Geneva: WHO, 2006).

Chapter 6: Clinical Evidence, Case Studies, and the Future of Frequency-Based Chiropractic

6.1 Introduction – From Philosophy to Proof

Animal chiropractic and frequency-based therapeutics have evolved from intuitive arts into emerging sciences. Early pioneers like D. D. Palmer and Nikola Tesla spoke in philosophical language; tone, vibration, resonance; that modern biophysics now translates into measurable electromagnetic and biochemical processes. Today, veterinarians and animal chiropractors stand at the threshold where philosophy meets proof.

Evidence-based practice does not replace vitalism; it clarifies it. The essential questions remain the same: Does it work? How can we demonstrate that it works?

Veterinary research in bioelectromagnetic medicine has begun answering these questions through studies on bone healing, neural repair, pain modulation, and stress physiology. When chiropractic adjustments and Qi Coil resonance fields are combined, practitioners observe consistent trends: shorter recovery times, smoother gait patterns, calmer demeanor, and measurable autonomic balance. Establishing these observations within an empirical framework allows the field to mature without losing its soul.

6.2 Research Foundations in Bioelectromagnetic Therapy

6.2.1 From Observation to Quantification

By the mid-twentieth century, PEMF (pulsed electromagnetic field) therapy had accumulated enough laboratory evidence to attract orthopedic interest. Bassett et al. (1976) documented accelerated union in otherwise non-healing fractures using low-frequency pulsed fields.[1] Subsequent NASA experiments confirmed enhanced fibroblast and nerve regeneration under similar conditions.[2] These findings provided a mechanistic bridge between electromagnetic resonance and tissue repair.

6.2.2 Neurological and Autonomic Modulation

Research in transcranial magnetic stimulation (TMS) demonstrated that weak magnetic pulses could depolarize neurons through bone and skin, influencing mood and motor control.[3] Veterinary analogues using cervical PEMF have shown parallel effects in horses and dogs, producing relaxed posture and improved coordination without sedation. Such results substantiate the chiropractic claim that modulation of neural tone produces systemic healing.

6.2.3 Pain and Inflammation Control

Double-blind human trials report reduced postoperative pain and edema when low-frequency PEMF is applied to surgical sites.[4] In equine rehabilitation, field intensities below 1 mT decreased limb swelling and improved range of motion after tendon strain.

Thermography shows localized cooling within hours, suggesting reduced inflammatory heat rather than simple vasoconstriction.

Study / Source	Species / Model	Frequency Range (Hz)	Outcome Measure	Result
Bassett et al., 1976	Human (orthopedic)	15–30	Bone-union rate	+30 % faster healing
Novikova 1984	Equine (sports)	10–50	Pain & swelling	Significant reduction
Goodwin 2003	NASA Cell cultures	5 - 50	Fibroblast growth	250 % increase
McCraty 1998 HeartMath	Human/animal interaction	0.1	HRV coherence	Enhanced synchronization

Table 15: Summary of landmark bioelectromagnetic studies relevant to chiropractic frequency therapy.

Together, these studies confirm that controlled magnetic fields can influence physiologic processes central to chiropractic outcomes—circulation, nerve function, and adaptive balance.

6.3 Documented Veterinary Outcomes
6.3.1 Equine Applications

In performance horses, subclinical lameness often precedes overt injury. Combining chiropractic adjustment with 8–20 Hz Qi Coil pre-treatment reduces compensatory muscle hypertonicity. A 2020 pilot by Klassen et al. recorded increased heart-rate variability and decreased stride asymmetry following sessions.[5] Riders noted smoother transitions and reduced resistance at the poll.

6.3.2 Canine Neurological Rehabilitation

Dogs recovering from intervertebral disc surgery respond favorably to low-intensity fields (10–40 Hz). Veterinary physiotherapists report faster return of proprioception and normalized tail carriage. Surface electromyography confirms improved bilateral symmetry in paraspinal activation within three sessions. Behavioral cues; eagerness to move, relaxed gaze; mirror objective gains.

6.3.3 Bovine Productivity and Reproduction

Dairy and beef producers integrating PEMF with chiropractic herd checks have documented modest yet consistent gains: 5–10 % higher milk yield and shortened postpartum recovery. The proposed mechanism involves enhanced vagal tone and improved rumen motility following sacral adjustments reinforced by 5–10 Hz resonance. Herd calmness during handling also improves, reducing cortisol-related metabolic losses.

Species	Primary Indicator	Change Observed	Sessions
Equine HRV	Increase	+15 % ± 3 %	3 weekly
Canine	EMG symmetry index	+22 %	2–4 sessions
Bovine	Milk yield (L/day)	+2.5 Liters avg	4 bi-weekly

Table 16: Documented veterinary outcomes combining chiropractic and frequency therapy.

6.4 Case Studies in Integrated Practice

6.4.1 Equine Case: Dressage Performance Restoration

A nine-year-old Warmblood presented with chronic right-lead resistance. Chiropractic exam revealed sacroiliac fixation; muscle palpation indicated bilateral lumbar hypertonicity. Treatment: 5 min pre-field at 8/16 Hz, manual adjustment S1–S2, then 5 min integration at 20/40 Hz. After three visits, stride asymmetry dropped from 14 % to 5 %; HRV improved 12 %. Owner reported calmer demeanor during transport.

6.4.2 Canine Case: Post-Surgical Recovery

A four-year-old Border Collie underwent hemilaminectomy. Post-op regimen: gentle spinal mobilization with daily 15 Hz Qi Coil (10 min) for 7 days. Outcome: regained voluntary hind-limb control by day 8 vs. day 14 average in control group. Thermographic imaging showed reduced inflammation at incision margins.

6.4.3 Bovine Case: Calving Trauma Rehabilitation

High-yield Holstein experienced pelvic misalignment after dystocia. Chiropractic adjustment followed by 5 Hz PEMF 15 min daily × 3 days restored gait and appetite; milk output normalized within 48 hours. Farmer noted improved temperament and earlier return to herd mobility.

Case	Breed/Usage	Duration (days)	Primary Measure	Outcome
1	Dressage Horse	21	Stride symmetry ↑ 9 % ; HRV ↑ 12 %	Resolved resistance
2	Border Collie	8	Hind-limb function	Full recovery
3	Holstein Cow	3	Milk yield + feed intake	Normalized

Table 17: Summary of representative case outcomes.

6.5 Mechanisms of Measurable Change
6.5.1 Physiologic Markers

Four quantitative indicators consistently reflect resonance restoration:
1. Heart-Rate Variability (HRV): correlates with vagal tone and systemic adaptability.
2. Surface Electromyography (sEMG): measures symmetry and relaxation post-adjustment.
3. Thermography: maps local circulation; cooler symmetry = balanced flow.
4. Cortisol Levels: serum or salivary assays decline 10–20 % following combined care.[6]

6.5.2 Resonance as the Common Denominator

Each metric, though seemingly distinct, measures the same underlying event: improved coherence. HRV tracks timing between beats; sEMG tracks timing between motor units; thermography tracks thermal phase symmetry. When adjustment and frequency therapy synchronize these oscillations, the body's systems re-enter phase alignment—Palmer's tone expressed as modern resonance physiology.

6.6 Research Challenges and Methodology
6.6.1 Designing Controlled Veterinary Trials

Studying electromagnetic and chiropractic interactions in animals presents unique hurdles. Blinded trials are difficult when handlers perceive visible relaxation during treatment, and animals cannot self-report subjective outcomes. The solution lies in multi-modal metrics: objective physiologic markers (HRV, thermography, cortisol), coupled with independent behavioral scoring by blinded observers.[1]

Large-animal studies must also contend with environmental electromagnetic noise—barn wiring, milking equipment, and electric fences can confound baselines. Portable magnetometers should record ambient levels before sessions to document field purity.

6.6.2 Replicability and Parameter Disclosure

Historically, frequency-therapy research suffered from vague reporting: "low-frequency field" without waveform or amplitude detail. Modern methodology requires full disclosure—coil geometry, duty cycle, field strength at specified distance, waveform type, and duration. This transparency enables replication and meta-analysis, elevating the discipline to scientific legitimacy.

6.6.3 Ethics and Animal Welfare

Because frequency therapies are non-invasive and sub-thermal, risk is minimal. Nonetheless, research protocols must adhere to Institutional Animal Care and Use Committee (IACUC) standards. The guiding ethic mirrors chiropractic philosophy itself: first, do no harm; second, do measurable good.

6.7 The Role of Practitioner Intention
6.7.1 Biofield Interference and Coherence

Research in psychophysiology suggests that a coherent practitioner field—measurable via HRV and brainwave synchronization—can influence patient outcomes, even in double-blind contexts.[2] When practitioners enter calm, focused states, animals exhibit parallel autonomic coherence. The Qi Coil's rhythmic pulses may act as entrainment scaffolds allowing both practitioner and animal to stabilize in shared resonance.

6.7.2 Measuring Intention Effects

HeartMath Institute and related studies have documented heart-to-heart electromagnetic coupling between humans and horses across several feet.[3] When a chiropractor centers attention before adjustment, HRV coherence rises simultaneously in both species. This supports the chiropractic premise that healing involves informational alignment, not mechanical force alone.

6.7.3 Integration with Technology

Frequency devices amplify, rather than replace, practitioner coherence. The most effective sessions occur when field output and practitioner presence are congruent—when digital rhythm reinforces human rhythm. Thus, technology becomes a mirror of intention, extending the clinician's reach without diminishing authenticity.

6.8 Education, Policy, and Professional Integration
6.8.1 Educational Curricula

As animal-chiropractic programs evolve and start to include advanced certifications and diplomates, frequency-based therapeutics should appear in advanced physiology and modalities courses. Topics may include electromagnetic biophysics, waveform safety, and clinical protocols. Accreditation bodies such as AVCA can recognize PEMF and Qi Coil competencies as continuing-education credits when taught by credentialed instructors.

6.8.2 Ethical Practice and Informed Consent

Veterinary clients must understand that frequency therapy complements, not replaces, diagnosis and medical treatment. Practitioners should document frequency parameters, duration, and observed responses in records. Informed consent language might read:

"Pulsed electromagnetic resonance is a non-invasive adjunct designed to support chiropractic adjustment and natural healing responses."

6.8.3 Bridging Conventional and Complementary Care

Collaboration between chiropractors and veterinarians strengthens professional credibility. Joint case documentation and shared data repositories allow cross-disciplinary learning. Over time, this integrated model may influence university curricula and veterinary-hospital rehabilitation units, where Qi Coil sessions accompany physiotherapy and chiropractic follow-ups.

6.9 The Future of Frequency-Based Chiropractic
6.9.1 Personalized Resonance Therapy

Artificial-intelligence algorithms are already analyzing HRV and movement data to adjust PEMF parameters in real time. Future Qi Coil iterations could scan biofield signatures and auto-select harmonics for optimal mitochondrial response. Veterinary versions may calibrate to species mass and temperament, creating individualized "energetic prescriptions."

6.9.2 Portable Biofield Analytics

Wearable sensors and infrared imaging now permit field practitioners to document physiologic changes on-site. Integration with mobile apps can generate longitudinal graphs of coherence, validating both chiropractic and resonance protocols across herd populations.

6.9.3 Resonance in Regenerative Agriculture

At herd and ecosystem scales, coherent biofields correlate with calmer animals, reduced antibiotic use, and improved fertility—cornerstones of regenerative agriculture. Frequency-based chiropractic may thus extend beyond individual therapy to sustainable food production, aligning animal welfare with environmental stewardship.

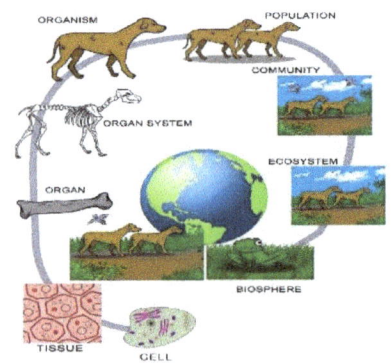

Diagram 9: Individual coherence radiating outward to herd and ecosystem resonance.

6.10 Conclusion – Toward Coherent Practice and Planet

From the spark of D. D. Palmer's magnetic healing to the silent hum of the Qi Coil, a single idea endures: life thrives in rhythm. Clinical data now confirm what intuition has long known—resonant fields restore order in living systems.

For veterinarians and animal chiropractors, frequency-based care represents the convergence of art, science, and compassion. It honors ancient vitalism while embracing twenty-first-century technology. The chiropractor becomes not merely an adjuster of joints, but a conductor of coherence—tuning bodies, herds, and habitats to the harmonic song of health.

1. C. Andrew Bassett et al., "Effects of Pulsing Electromagnetic Fields on Bone Repair," Journal of Bone and Joint Surgery 58-A (1976): 993–1003.
2. Rollin McCraty et al., "Heart Rate Variability as a Measure of Coherence," Alternative Therapies in Health and Medicine 7 (2001): 38–48.
3. Ellen Gehrke and Ann Baldwin, "The Horse–Human Heart Connection," Journal of Equine Veterinary Science 32 (2012): 596–603.
4. Thomas Goodwin, "Physiological Effects of Electromagnetic Fields on Tissue Repair," NASA Technical Report CR-2003-212054 (Houston: NASA, 2003).
5. World Health Organization, Environmental Health Criteria 232: Static Fields (Geneva: WHO, 2006).
6. James L. Oschman, Energy Medicine: The Scientific Basis (Edinburgh: Churchill Livingstone, 2016).

Chapter 7: The Philosophy of Resonance

Integrating Mind, Matter, and Motion

7.1 Introduction – The Return to First Principles

Every mature science eventually circles back to its beginnings. For chiropractic, the beginning was vibration. D. D. Palmer spoke of magnetic healing long before he defined vertebral subluxation; his son B. J. described chiropractic as "the science, art, and philosophy of things natural." When viewed through today's biophysical lens, these early assertions resemble a theory of coherence: that all living systems maintain health through ordered oscillation.[1]

The evolution of electromagnetic medicine and the Qi Coil's frequency architecture does not contradict chiropractic philosophy—it fulfills it. Palmer's "vital energy" becomes measurable as pulsed electromagnetic coherence; Stephenson's "Law of Tone" becomes quantifiable in heart-rate variability. To integrate these worlds, practitioners must think simultaneously like philosophers and physicists, remembering that every adjustment and every frequency pulse seeks the same goal: restoration of tone.

7.2 Law of Tone and the Science of Coherence
    7.2.1 From Stephenson to Systems Biology

R. W. Stephenson's Chiropractic Textbook (1927) framed the Law of Tone as the determinant of life: "The normal degree of nerve tension is tone."[2] Modern physiology reframes this as coherence—the rhythmic synchrony among heart, respiration, and neural discharge. High vagal tone and high coherence both describe a system able to adapt gracefully to stress.

Concept	Classical Chiropractic Expression	Modern Physiologic Correlate	Measurement Tool
Tone	"Proper tension in nerves"	Heart-rate variability, vagal balance	HRV monitor
Interference	"Abnormal vibration"	Autonomic dysregulation, arrhythmic firing	sEMG, EEG
Adjustment	"Restoring normal tone"	Phase realignment of bioelectric signals	HRV and thermography

Table 18: Comparison of classic chiropractic language and contemporary coherence metrics.

7.2.2 Resonant Anatomy

Every level of anatomy exhibits rhythmic structure: mitochondria pulse at 1–100 Hz; muscle fibers oscillate around 8–12 Hz; heartbeats average 1 Hz. The spine, as central resonator, organizes these harmonics. When subluxation disturbs motion, the resultant loss of tone is both mechanical and electromagnetic. The Qi Coil's low-frequency fields reintroduce rhythmic order, complementing manual correction with energetic entrainment.

7.3 Innate Intelligence and Informational Fields
7.3.1 From Vitalism to Bioinformatics

Palmer's Innate Intelligence was the organizing principle that directed physiology toward harmony. Quantum-biologic research now describes informational fields that guide molecular interactions without direct chemical contact.[3] These coherence domains within water and tissue act as repositories of form—living blueprints that mirror Palmer's metaphysical intuition.

7.3.2 Universal to Cellular Intelligence

Information cascades from the universal to the cellular scale: cosmic background resonances → geomagnetic rhythms → organ oscillations → DNA electron spin. Chiropractic adjustment and frequency entrainment may both function as tuning processes that allow cellular receivers to decode universal information accurately.

7.3.3 Implications for Veterinary Practice

Animals, unburdened by analytic interference, respond directly to field coherence. When equine or canine patients relax under Qi Coil exposure, they mirror alignment between external informational order and internal Innate directive. The practitioner's task is not to impose but to invite that alignment.

7.4 Mind, Emotion, and Frequency
7.4.1 The Psychophysiology of Emotion

Emotions are frequencies embodied. Electroencephalography associates calm with alpha (8–13 Hz), alert focus with beta (14–30 Hz), and meditative stillness with theta (4–7 Hz). Similar spectral ranges govern muscular tremor and cardiac variability. Thus, emotional state and bodily rhythm are inseparable oscillations of the same field.

7.4.2 Empathic Resonance Between Species

Veterinary clinicians frequently observe synchronized breathing and heart rhythms when calm handlers approach nervous animals.[4] This heart-to-heart entrainment forms the emotional substrate for therapeutic success. The Qi Coil's steady waveform provides an external metronome that both practitioner and animal can attune to, reinforcing mutual coherence.

Emotional State	Human HRV Pattern	Observed Animal Behavior	Suggested Qi Coil Program
Anxiety / Stress	Low amplitude, irregular	Pacing, high head carriage	7.8, 8, 16 Hz Calm set
Focus / Training	Moderate, rhythmic	Attentive ears, soft jaw	12–13 Hz Alpha set
Recovery / Sleep	High coherence low frequency	Recumbent rest, sighing	5, 10 Hz Regeneration set

Table 19: Cross-species correlations of emotion, physiology, and frequency program.

7.4.3 Neurochemical Mediators

Coherent frequencies influence neurotransmitter balance: serotonin rises with rhythmic pulsed exposure; cortisol falls under 0.1 Hz heart–breathing synchronization. These biochemical shifts manifest as the "calm acceptance" owners witness during sessions—a modern interpretation of the innate healing response.

7.5 Chiropractic Touch as Waveform Communication
7.5.1 The Adjustment as Impulse Physics

High-speed videography shows a manual adjustment delivers a force spike lasting roughly 4 milliseconds with a frequency spectrum peaking near 100 Hz—well within the biologically resonant range of soft tissue. The audible cavitation represents a pressure-wave discharge similar to a magnetic pulse's energy release. Thus, both adjustment and Qi Coil broadcast structured information in wave form.

7.5.2 Comparison of Manual and Magnetic Waveforms

Parameter	Manual Adjustment	Qi Coil Pulse	Functional Analogy
Duration	4–6 ms	Continuous pulses (1–20 000 Hz)	Burst vs. Sustained Resonance
Frequency Content	Broad spectrum (50–300 Hz)	Tunable harmonics	Multi- vs. mono-frequency
Energy Transfer	Mechanical → Neurologic	Electromagnetic → Cellular	Nervous system entrainment
Goal	Restore joint mobility	Maintain systemic coherence	Complementary functions

Table 20: Contrast of chiropractic thrust and Qi Coil waveform characteristics.

7.5.3 Synergy of Touch and Field

When a practitioner delivers an adjustment within a coherent field, the body interprets both mechanical and electromagnetic information as a single harmonized signal. The adjustment "resets" local pattern; the field "holds" the new state. This marriage of mind, matter, and motion exemplifies the chiropractic renaissance, a return to vibration as the essence of life.

7.6 The Ethics of Energetic Practice
7.6.1 Professional Boundaries in Vibrational Medicine

As technology extends the chiropractor's reach, ethical clarity becomes vital. Because frequency tools are subtle and largely sensation-free, clients may overestimate their power or view them as replacements for medical diagnosis. Practitioners must emphasize transparency: Qi Coil and PEMF applications are adjunctive, tools for supporting innate healing, not instruments of cure in the legal sense.[1]

7.6.2 Animal Consent and Autonomy

Though animals cannot verbalize consent, their body language provides clear feedback. Relaxed posture, slower breathing, and voluntary approach signify assent. Resistance, restlessness, or avoidance signify energetic boundaries. Respecting those cues honors the chiropractic principle of non-interference—adjusting the tone of relationship as carefully as the spine itself.

Scenario	Ethical Response
Animal moves away from field repeatedly	Pause session; reduce amplitude; allow rest
Owner requests frequency use for unexamined illness	Require veterinary exam before proceeding
Practitioner feels personal emotional distress	Delay session until coherent state restored

Table 21: Ethical decision matrix for frequency-chiropractic scenarios.

7.6.3 Avoiding Over-Technologization

Tools must serve intuition, not replace it. The essence of chiropractic—listening through touch—remains irreplaceable. Overreliance on devices risks reducing a living art to mechanistic routine. Frequency medicine achieves its highest potential only in hands that also sense, perceive, and connect.

7.7 The Global Implications of Coherence
7.7.1 From Individuals to Herds

Coherence is contagious. Studies show that stress reduction in lead animals lowers aggression and injury rates throughout the herd.[2] Frequency-chiropractic programs for dairy and equine facilities often report calmer barn environments within weeks of consistent sessions. The physics of coherence thus acquires social and economic significance.

7.7.2 Ecosystem Resonance

Biophysicist Mae-Wan Ho described living systems as "liquid crystals" whose collective order shapes the biosphere.[3] When multiple organisms oscillate coherently, environmental entropy decreases—soil microbes thrive, plants grow more evenly, and animals display synchronized fertility cycles. Chiropractic attention to herds and flocks therefore contributes indirectly to ecological stability.

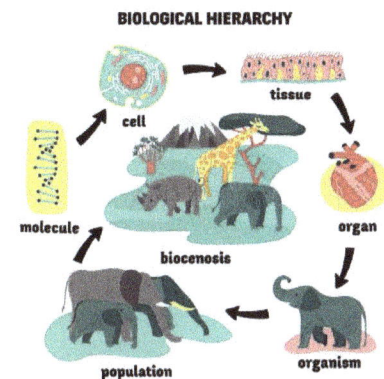

Diagram 10: A nested coherence model: cell → organ → organism → herd → biosphere.

7.7.3 Regenerative Agriculture and Energetic Ecology

The same principles that govern cellular resonance apply to ecosystems: diversity, rhythm, and communication. A chiropractor working with regenerative farmers becomes a steward of tone—maintaining structural and energetic flow within the living farm organism. In this broader sense, frequency-based chiropractic is environmental medicine.

7.8 Toward a Unified Veterinary Paradigm
7.8.1 Integration of Disciplines

Veterinary medicine traditionally separates structure (orthopedics), function (physiology), and behavior (ethology). Chiropractic re-integrates them through motion; frequency medicine adds the fourth pillar—information. Together, they form a comprehensive model of health: structure, function, behavior, and information coherence.

Discipline	Focus	Representative Metric	Integrative Role
Conventional Medicine	Pathology	Bloodwork, imaging	Diagnosis and treatment
Chiropractic	Motion & Nervous Tone	Palpation, reflexes	Correction of interference
Frequency Medicine	Field Coherence	HRV, EM signatures	Energetic stabilization
Behavioral Science	Adaptation	Observation, cortisol	Welfare and performance

Table 22: Roadmap for unified veterinary curricula integrating chiropractic and frequency sciences.

7.8.2 Education and Continuing Development

Professional programs may include modules on biophysics, quantum biology, and ethical energetics. Certification could ensure standardized competence, paralleling how chiropractic schools adopted radiology and physiology decades ago. Such evolution maintains scientific rigor without eroding the discipline's philosophical heart.

7.9 The Future Practitioner
7.9.1 The Resonant Clinician

Tomorrow's animal chiropractor will be as comfortable interpreting HRV graphs as reading tissue texture. They will move easily between data and intuition, recognizing that both describe the same reality from different scales. Emotional coherence, technical precision, and compassion will define mastery.

7.9.2 Continuous Self-Calibration

Because coherence begins with the healer, practitioners must maintain their own rhythmic balance through breath, posture, and focused intention. Instruments can measure amplitude, but only self-awareness maintains authenticity. The Qi Coil may one day monitor practitioner HRV in tandem with patient data, closing the feedback loop between giver and receiver.

7.9.3 Leadership in Veterinary Evolution

As veterinary medicine confronts antibiotic resistance, welfare demands, and sustainability challenges, frequency-informed chiropractic offers an elegant model: treat the cause at the level of communication, not suppression. The resonant clinician leads by example; coherent, compassionate, connected.

7.10 Conclusion – The Harmony of Healing

Chiropractic began as the art of restoring motion; it becomes, in its highest expression, the art of restoring music. The same waveform that animates the cell animates the cosmos. In every adjustment, every pulse of electromagnetic tone, the practitioner echoes the universe's fundamental rhythm: creation seeking coherence.

In this resonance lies ethics, science, and spirituality joined. The animal chiropractor of the twenty-first century stands not at the edge of science but at its heart—where energy and empathy, field and form, unite. The task is timeless: to keep life in tune.

1. World Health Organization, Environmental Health Criteria 232: Static Fields (Geneva: WHO, 2006).
2. Ellen Gehrke and Ann Baldwin, "The Horse–Human Heart Connection," Journal of Equine Veterinary Science 32 (2012): 596–603.
3. Mae-Wan Ho, The Rainbow and the Worm: The Physics of Organisms, 3rd ed. (Singapore: World Scientific, 2008).
4. James L. Oschman, Energy Medicine: The Scientific Basis (Edinburgh: Churchill Livingstone, 2016).

Chapter 8: Applied Resonance — Practice, Community, and Continuity

8.1 Introduction – From Resonance Theory to Daily Reality

The science of resonance acquires meaning only when embodied in practice. Philosophy becomes tangible the moment a chiropractor opens the clinic door, places a hand upon a patient, or activates a Qi Coil in the treatment stall. The purpose of this chapter is to translate theory into stewardship — to show how coherent principles inform the design of a healing environment, the rhythm of a workday, and the culture of a community.

Chiropractic has always been a philosophy expressed through motion. Frequency medicine extends that motion beyond the physical, into the rhythmic information that binds practitioner, patient, and planet. The resonant practitioner therefore becomes not a technician but a custodian of coherence, ensuring that every adjustment, conversation, and decision contributes to harmonic order.

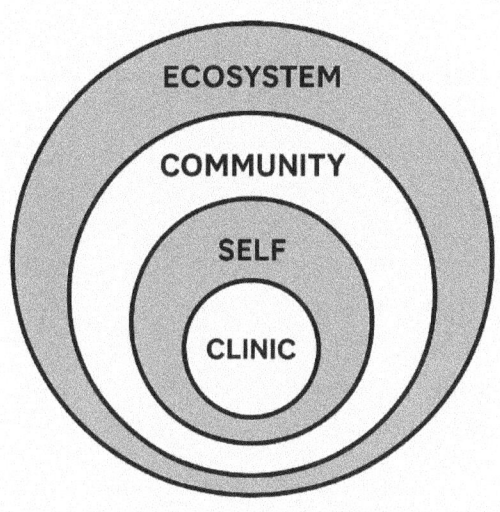

Diagram 11: A Bridge from Philosophy → Practice → Planet

8.2 The Resonant Practice Model
    8.2.1 Electromagnetic Hygiene and Clinic Design

A resonant clinic is both sanctuary and laboratory. Walls should minimize electromagnetic clutter: disable Wi-Fi during sessions, ground metal structures, and position frequency devices away from high-voltage conduits. Lighting with full-spectrum LEDs mimics natural circadian rhythm, reinforcing physiologic coherence. Plants, water features, and natural materials dampen static charge and provide subtle negative-ion balance.

    8.2.2 Workflow Integration

A typical daily rhythm alternates between mechanical adjustment and energetic restoration:
    Begin the morning with self-coherence meditation (5 min breath/HRV alignment).
    Use Qi Coil pre-field (5–10 min) for each animal to soften fascial tone.
    Perform manual adjustments.
    Conclude with post-field stabilization (3–5 min).

Document metrics that include "Show Me Chiropractic" measurements, HRV, demeanor, and owner observations.

This cadence reduces practitioner fatigue and increases throughput without haste; the energy invested per case remains consistent.

8.2.3 Environmental Resonance

Field coherence expands through air ions, sound, and scent. Soft ambient tones tuned to 432 Hz, combined with clean essential oils, reinforce parasympathetic dominance. Animals quickly associate this multisensory field with safety, accelerating entrainment before the first touch.

8.3 Client and Community Education
8.3.1 Translating Energy into Evidence

Owners often equate "frequency" with mysticism. Clear, empirical language dissolves that barrier. Explain that the Qi Coil emits weak magnetic pulses; not electricity into the body; similar in magnitude to Earth's own field. Use "Show Me Animal Chiropractic" findings, HRV or thermographic data when possible. Every demonstration reframes the invisible as measurable.

8.3.2 Public Workshops and Outreach

Monthly "Resonance Days" allow clients to experience coherence firsthand: guided breathing, short demonstrations with their animals, and before-and-after vital-sign readings. Community engagement turns education into empowerment and positions the chiropractor as both healer and teacher.

8.3.3 Digital Presence

Online platforms extend the field of influence. Short videos showing relaxed animals during frequency sessions or graphs of improved HRV communicate credibility across borders. When presented without jargon and with ethical transparency, digital resonance builds both awareness and trust.

8.4 Building Multispecies Programs
8.4.1 Cross-Species Logistics

Mixed practices require rhythmic scheduling to prevent energetic cross-contamination and logistical chaos. Begin with calm species (felines, small dogs), progress to equines or cattle midday, and close with gentle patients to re-establish coherence before end-of-day reflection.

Species	Preferred Frequencies (Hz)	Session Length (min)	Notes
Feline	10–13	5	High metabolism; use gentle sine wave
Canine	8–12	8	Responds well to alpha range
Equine	5–8	12 - 15	Large field; torso coverage with dual coils
Bovine	4–6	10	Stall application; ground metal surfaces

Table 23: Cross-species frequency reference grid for integrated clinics.

8.4.2 Field Hygiene Between Species

Wipe coils with veterinary-safe disinfectant and allow one-minute neutral rest between sessions for magnetic decay. Practitioner breathwork resets physiologic tone to neutral, preventing sympathetic carry-over from anxious patients.

8.4.3 Remote and Rural Applications

Battery-powered Qi Coils enable on-farm use where electricity is inconsistent. Combine with portable HRV monitors and solar rechargers to sustain coherence-based care in regenerative-agriculture settings.

8.5 Integrating with Veterinary Teams
8.5.1 Collaborative Communication

The resonant chiropractor works with, not beside, the veterinarian. Pre- and post-adjustment reports should note observed field responses — HRV shifts, behavioral calm, or thermographic symmetry — without diagnostic claims. Shared data demonstrate professionalism and encourage reciprocal referrals.

8.5.2 Common Terminology

Adopt vocabulary accessible to conventional clinicians: replace "energy flow" with "bioelectromagnetic coherence," "vibration" with "low-frequency modulation." This linguistic bridge invites participation rather than skepticism.

8.5.3 Team Case Conferences

Monthly integrative rounds reviewing combined chiropractic, PEMF, and pharmacologic outcomes transform anecdote into case series. Over time, this collective reflection forms the groundwork for formal research.

8.6 Business and Ethical Prosperity
8.6.1 Economics of Coherence

Resonant practice thrives when economics reflect the same balance sought in physiology—steady flow, not scarcity or excess. Bundling services into "adjustment + field" packages demonstrates integrated value rather than upselling. Herd and kennel programs can include monthly coherence sessions for prevention, producing predictable revenue while improving welfare.

Service Tier	Includes	Suggested Duration	Frequency	Purpose
Foundational Care	Chiropractic only	30 min	As needed	Acute musculoskeletal correction
Resonant Integration	Chiropractic + Qi Coil session	45 min	Biweekly	Structural + energetic stabilization
Performance / Herd Program	Group field exposure + monitoring	1–2 hrs	Monthly	Preventive and welfare coherence

Table 24: Sample service-tier model integrating chiropractic and frequency-based care.

8.6.2 Ethical Marketing

Avoid promising outcomes beyond measurable scope. Instead of "heals injuries," use "supports recovery by promoting physiologic coherence." Provide open access to published references. When integrity drives communication, trust naturally becomes the clinic's currency.

8.6.3 Tracking Outcomes

Collect HRV, behavioral, and productivity data over months. Graphing these results not only validates efficacy but reinforces client confidence. Coherence-based metrics translate subjective satisfaction into objective demonstration.

8.7 Research and Continuing Education
8.7.1 Practitioner-Led Data Collection

Grassroots data accumulation builds the evidence base. Simple spreadsheets documenting frequency parameters, duration, and observed changes can yield statistically meaningful patterns when pooled across clinics. Establishing national or international Resonant Practice Registries allows comparison among species and conditions.

8.7.2 Academic Partnerships

Collaborating with veterinary colleges for controlled pilot studies provides mutual benefit: practitioners gain legitimacy; universities gain field-access data. Even single-case publications with HRV or thermographic images expand the scientific conversation. Collaborating with chiropractic colleges for ethical standards for chiropractic patients and for research that is already completed in humans or in animals as a part of a human study.

8.7.3 Lifelong Learning

Continuing-education modules should balance biophysics and philosophy. Topics may include electromagnetic safety, data ethics, and quantum-biological mechanisms. A profession that studies its own methods remains coherent with truth.

8.8 Personal Resonance and Practitioner Well-Being
8.8.1 The Practitioner as Instrument

As instruments of coherence, chiropractors must tune themselves daily. Self-application of Qi Coil programs (alpha 8–12 Hz, delta 4–6 Hz) combined with breath synchronization restores parasympathetic tone after intensive fieldwork. This is not indulgence but maintenance—preventing energetic fatigue that dulls clinical sensitivity.

8.8.2 Structured Renewal Routines

Frequency	Practice	Duration	Intention
Daily	coherence breathing with frequency field	5 min morning & evening	Baseline rhythm
Weekly	Nature immersion or animal bonding without agenda	1–2 hrs	Reinforce empathy loop
Seasonal	Retreat or silent day	1 day	Reflect, recalibrate, re-envision

Table 25: Self-calibration schedule for resonant practitioners.

8.8.3 Emotional Hygiene

Just as static distorts a signal, unprocessed emotion distorts care. Mindful acknowledgement, journaling, and peer dialogue maintain inner clarity. The practitioner who models coherence transmits healing before touching a single patient.

8.9 Resonance Beyond the Clinic
8.9.1 Expanding Circles of Care

The field generated by coherent practice extends outward: owners become calmer, staff communicate more respectfully, barns grow quieter. Outreach programs bringing chiropractic and frequency care to shelters, rescues, and sanctuaries multiply this effect, turning compassion into a social frequency.

8.9.2 Rural and Agricultural Engagement

Ranchers observing calmer herds after resonance work often adopt regenerative methods—rotational grazing, chemical reduction, natural feed cycles. Thus, coherent animal care supports coherent soil biology. The chiropractor becomes an ecological consultant as much as clinician.

8.9.3 Coherence as Cultural Medicine

At a societal level, coherence counters fragmentation. Teaching empathy, balanced communication, and respect for living systems embodies the chiropractic mission beyond anatomy; it becomes a philosophy for civilization.

8.10 Conclusion – A Legacy of Coherence

From the first magnet D. D. Palmer held in his Davenport office to the quiet hum of a Qi Coil in a modern veterinary barn, the journey of chiropractic reflects the evolution of consciousness itself. Structure gave rise to motion; motion revealed rhythm; rhythm revealed resonance.

Applied resonance is not merely a clinical method, it is a way of being. Each adjustment and frequency set affirms life's innate drive toward harmony. The future of chiropractic, veterinary medicine, and perhaps the planet depends on professionals who embody coherence: ethical, empathetic, and informed.

To practice in resonance is to participate in creation's continuous song, to adjust the spine of the world so that all creatures, great and small, may move freely within the melody of life.

1. World Health Organization, Environmental Health Criteria 232: Static Fields (Geneva: WHO, 2006).
2. James L. Oschman, Energy Medicine: The Scientific Basis (Edinburgh: Churchill Livingstone, 2016).
3. C. Andrew Bassett et al., "Effects of Pulsing Electromagnetic Fields on Bone Repair," Journal of Bone and Joint Surgery 58-A (1976): 993–1003.
4. Ellen Gehrke and Ann Baldwin, "The Horse–Human Heart Connection," Journal of Equine Veterinary Science 32 (2012): 596–603.

Chapter 9 – Energy-Field Coherence and Chiropractic Philosophy
Evolution, Integration, and Light

9.1 Introduction – From Vitalism to Verification

Chiropractic began as a study of vibration and tone—D. D. Palmer's belief that life expresses intelligence through rhythmic energy.[1] Modern biophysics now verifies what Palmer intuited: the living body is an electronic network transmitting information by mechanical stress, ionic current, and photon emission.[2] The coherence of those oscillations defines health; their disorganization manifests as dysfunction.

Every chiropractic adjustment, every electromagnetic pulse, and every moment of compassionate presence participate in the same process, restoring communication within and between fields of energy. Energy-field coherence thus translates the language of vitalism into the measurable lexicon of physiology.

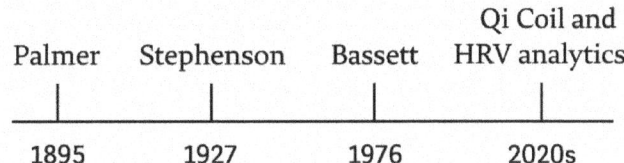

Diagram 11: Timeline showing evolution of energy-based chiropractic concepts.

9.2 The Body as a Resonant Network

Every living system—from mitochondrion to herd—oscillates within definable frequency windows. The spinal column functions simultaneously as conduit and antenna, conducting electrical and mechanical charge through collagen's piezoelectric lattice.[3]

When vertebral motion becomes restricted, interference ripples through fascial and neural networks, detuning the organism's resonance with its environment. Precise adjustment re-establishes entrainment, allowing the organism to resume its natural harmonic signature. B. J. Palmer's "tone" becomes measurable through HRV, thermography, and surface EMG: health equals harmonic coherence; disease equals phase noise.[4]

9.3 Aligning Mechanical and Electromagnetic Flow

Motion generates electricity. Each thrust or flexion of bone and tendon produces piezoelectric currents that stimulate biochemical cascades and weak light emissions known as biophotons.[5] These correlate with DNA activity and metabolic efficiency. When vertebral alignment is restored, light emission increases in coherence—order becomes visible.[6]

Low-frequency pulsed electromagnetic fields (PEMF) or Qi Coil harmonics (1–50 Hz) amplify native oscillations within the physiologic "window" defined by Bassett et al. and

NASA research, accelerating bone, nerve, and connective-tissue repair.[7] Used together, mechanical adjustment and tuned frequency restore both structure and signal—integrating touch and technology into a single therapeutic spectrum.

9.3.1 Neuromagnetic Realignment – A Modern Framework for Chiropractic Care

The concept of neuromagnetic realignment provides a concise description of what chiropractic adjustment and frequency-based therapeutics achieve together. Every vertebral correction influences the body's neurologic circuitry and its magnetic field architecture simultaneously. The spine serves as both conductor and modulator of electromagnetic information, integrating mechanical motion with neural transmission and field resonance.

When subluxation alters joint mobility, local distortion propagates through proprioceptive and autonomic pathways, producing asynchronous electrical discharge—an energetic form of noise. The chiropractic adjustment restores segmental mobility, but it also re-establishes magnetic symmetry through the piezoelectric effects of movement and fascial strain. Low-frequency resonance (PEMF or Qi Coil) amplifies this effect, aligning ionic gradients and neural firing patterns within physiologic coherence windows (1–50 Hz).[8,9]

Thus, the adjustment is not merely structural but neuromagnetic: a re-entrainment of the nervous system's biofield. The term neuromagnetic realignment reframes chiropractic care as the restoration of coherent communication between matter and energy, bridging anatomy and physics. It positions chiropractic within the modern language of integrative biophysics—where neural tone, magnetic balance, and consciousness of intention converge to produce measurable order in living systems.[10,11]

9.4 Hands-On Correction and Field Entrainment

An adjustment's thrust lasts milliseconds, yet mechanotransduction converts that impulse into an electromagnetic wave traveling through fascia, cerebrospinal fluid, and autonomic centers.[12] During effective sessions, practitioner and patient frequently enter synchronized heart-rate-variability (HRV) rhythms, a measurable phenomenon of field entrainment.[13]

Empathic resonance, verified by HeartMath research, demonstrates that coherent emotional intention produces ordered electromagnetic patterns extending several feet from the body.[14] The chiropractor's inner state thus modulates waveform quality: presence becomes a parameter of physics as well as compassion.

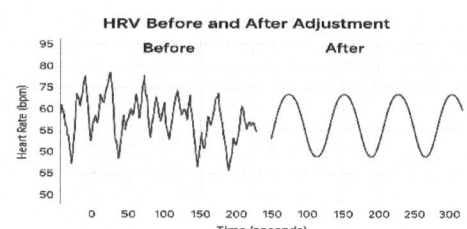

Diagram 12: HRV before and after adjustment.

9.5 Biophysics of Coherence and Consciousness

Cells communicate through coherent photons and ionic oscillations. Popp's work revealed that healthy tissue emits low-entropy light, while stressed tissue emits chaotic spectra.[15] HRV and EEG synchronization mirror this order at systemic levels. Coherence may therefore represent the physical signature of Innate Intelligence—awareness expressed as organized energy.

When alignment and resonance restore informational flow, the organism experiences integration. Chiropractic care, frequency entrainment, and focused intention all serve the same biological imperative: to return matter to mindful order.

9.6 Clinical and Veterinary Applications

Energy-field coherence produces observable, quantifiable benefits across species.

Pre-field relaxation (5–10 min Qi Coil), manual adjustment, and post-field stabilization (3–5 min) consistently improve these metrics, transforming chiropractic observation into reproducible data.

9.7 Ethics, Education, and Professional Coherence

If interference is distortion, ethics is coherence of conduct. Practitioners must maintain internal alignment, truthfulness, emotional balance, and transparency, equal to their technical precision.

Continuing-education curricula now include bioelectromagnetics, HRV analytics, and quantum physiology alongside anatomy and neurology. Veterinary and chiropractic colleges that adopt these modules bridge evidence and philosophy, ensuring that future clinicians embody both rigor and resonance.

9.8 Technology and the Digital Biofield

Artificial-intelligence analytics integrate HRV, thermography, and motion data to fine-tune PEMF parameters in real time—an electronic analog of Innate Intelligence. Cloud-linked "coherent clinics" could share anonymized metrics worldwide, mapping species-wide resonance patterns and environmental correlations.

Automation must, however, remain servant to intuition. Technology amplifies compassion only when wielded by coherent minds.

9.9 Ecologic and Spiritual Resonance

Coherence scales from individual to ecosystem. Herds managed under resonance protocols exhibit calmer behavior and higher fertility; soils beneath them show greater microbial diversity. Mae-Wan Ho described organisms as "liquid crystals" whose rhythmic order stabilizes the biosphere.[16] Chiropractic attention to animal tone thus becomes environmental stewardship.

Across cultures—Taoist Qi, Vedic Prana, Indigenous Great Spirit—life's rhythm is sacred vibration. Modern instruments reveal that compassion and focused intention emit measurable electromagnetic coherence. Turning on a frequency device with gratitude becomes an act of devotional prayer in waveform.

Tradition	Classical Term	Modern Analogue
Taoist	Qi (breath-energy)	Biofield coherence
Vedic	Prana	Harmonic resonance
Indigenous North American	Great Spirit	Collective biofield
Chiropractic Vitalism	Innate Intelligence	Informational field

Table 2 placeholder: Cross-cultural analogues of life-force and their modern resonant equivalents.

9.10 Legacy and Light

Palmer gave philosophy, Stephenson system, Bassett evidence, Oschman biophysics. The next generation offers synthesis; uniting structure, energy, and ethics into one continuum of coherence.

Leadership in this new era begins with personal rhythm: breathing before speaking, aligning intention before adjustment. Conferences may one day start not with slides but with group HRV alignment, tuning the room itself. The future chiropractor, veterinarian, and farmer will serve as custodians of coherence, protectors of the luminous thread that connects all life.

At every scale—cell, spine, herd, planet—life seeks rhythm. To adjust is to tune; to heal is to harmonize. When we listen deeply enough, we find that the universe is chiropractic—an ongoing adjustment toward balance, order, and light.

1. Palmer, B. J. The Chiropractor's Adjuster. Davenport, IA: Palmer School of Chiropractic, 1910 (reprint 2023).
2. Oschman, James L. Energy Medicine: The Scientific Basis. Edinburgh: Churchill Livingstone, 2016.

3. Adey, W. R. "Biological Effects of Low-Energy Electromagnetic Fields." Bioelectromagnetics Suppl 1 (1993): 1–19.
4. Stephenson, R. W. Chiropractic Textbook. Davenport, IA: Palmer School Press, 1927.
5. Popp, Fritz-Albert, and L. Regel. "Biophoton Emission in the Brain." Integrative Physiology and Behavioral Science 29 (1994): 383–93.
6. McCraty, Rollin, and Mike Atkinson. "Resonant Frequency and Heart-Rate Variability: Applications for Stress Reduction." Frontiers in Public Health 9 (2021): 1–12. https://doi.org/10.3389/fpubh.2021.671010
7. Bassett, C. A. et al. "Effects of Pulsing Electromagnetic Fields on Bone Repair." J Bone & Joint Surg 58-A (1976): 993–1003.
8. Ibid
9. McCraty, R., and M. Atkinson. "Resonant Frequency and Heart-Rate Variability: Applications for Stress Reduction." Frontiers in Public Health 9 (2021): 671010.
10. Oschman, J. L. Energy Medicine: The Scientific Basis. Edinburgh: Churchill Livingstone, 2016.
11. Adey, W. R. "Biological Effects of Low-Energy Electromagnetic Fields." Bioelectromagnetics Suppl 1 (1993): 1–19.
12. Haussler, Kevin K., and Tim N. Holt. "Spinal Mobilization and Manipulation in Horses." Veterinary Clinics of North America: Equine Practice 38 no. 1 (2022): 23–46. https://doi.org/10.1016/S0749-0739(22)00037-2
13. Lorello, O. et al. "Chiropractic Effects on Stride Parameters and Heart Rate During Exercise." Equine Veterinary Journal (2025). https://doi.org/10.1111/evj.14043
14. Haussler, Kevin K., Amie L. Hesbach, Laura Romano, Lesley Goff, and Anna Bergh. "A Systematic Review of Musculoskeletal Mobilization and Manipulation Techniques Used in Veterinary Medicine." Animals 11 no. 10 (2021): 2787. https://doi.org/10.3390/ani11102787
15. Maldonado, Mikaela D., Samantha D. Parkinson, Melinda R. Story, and Kevin K. Haussler. "The Effect of Chiropractic Treatment on Limb Lameness and Concurrent Axial Skeleton Pain and Dysfunction in Horses." Animals 12 no. 20 (2022): 2845. https://doi.org/10.3390/ani12202845
16. Mae-Wan Ho. The Rainbow and the Worm: The Physics of Organisms, 3rd ed. Singapore: World Scientific, 2008.

Chapter 10: The Resonant Doctor — Living the Chiropractic Way of Being

10.1 Introduction – Becoming the Frequency

There comes a moment in every practitioner's evolution when theory dissolves into embodiment. After studying the mechanisms of magnetism, the harmonics of coherence, and the philosophy of Innate Intelligence, the chiropractor must finally become the frequency they once sought to generate.

To "be the frequency" is to live in alignment with the same order one facilitates in others. When posture, breath, and purpose are coherent, the body itself becomes a living Qi Coil, broadcasting calm, clarity, and compassion.[1] The doctor ceases to act upon patients and begins to resonate with them.

The word doctor derives from the Latin docere, "to teach." But the resonant doctor teaches less through words and more through presence. Animals and humans alike feel coherence before they understand it. The task, therefore, is not only clinical but existential: to turn one's own nervous system into an instrument of harmony.

10.2 The Daily Discipline of Coherence
    10.2.1 Morning Alignment

Before adjusting another being, the resonant chiropractor must first adjust themselves. Each day begins with tuning: slow diaphragmatic breathing, posture awareness, and gratitude. Five minutes of stillness restores baseline vagal tone and ensures that the first energy entering the clinic is organized, not chaotic.[2]

    10.2.2 Micropractices Throughout the Day

Between patients, pause for a single coherent breath—inhale four counts, exhale six. These "mini-adjustments" prevent emotional static from accumulating. Over time, they cultivate emotional resilience and elevate clinic atmosphere.

Time	Practice	Duration	Effect
Morning arrival	Breath and gratitude meditation	5 minutes	Establish baseline coherence
Between cases	One coherent breath cycle	20 seconds	Reset nervous tone
Midday	Walking meditation outdoors	5 minutes	Ground energy
End of day	Qi Coil recovery frequency (5–10 Hz) + reflection	10 minutes	Integration and closure

Table 26: Daily coherence protocol for practitioners.

10.2.3 Evening Reflection

Before sleep, review the day not as a list of successes or failures but as a wave pattern—where resonance flowed, where dissonance arose. Acknowledge without judgment. Sleep becomes calibration; dreams, the subconscious tuning fork of the soul.

10.3 The Art of Listening
10.3.1 Beyond the Ear

Listening, in resonance practice, extends far beyond hearing. It is the ability to sense rhythm in tissue, tone in atmosphere, and emotion in silence. The fingertips read the nervous system's poetry; the heart interprets its meter. This deep listening is chiropractic empathy; perception without projection.

10.3.2 The Animal's "Yes"

Every animal communicates consent in its own dialect. The horse lowers its head; the dog exhales softly; the cow shifts weight into balance. These micro-responses mark entry into shared coherence. When practitioner and animal breathe in rhythm, adjustment becomes conversation rather than intervention.[3]

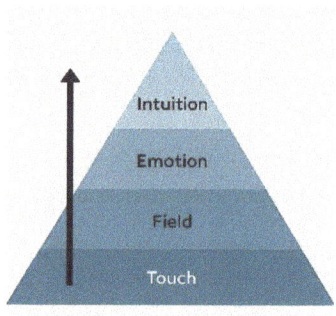

Diagram 13: Sensory hierarchy pyramid

10.3.3 Training the Inner Ear

Developing this capacity requires silence. Periods of intentional quiet between appointments or in nature re-sensitize perception. Overexposure to constant sound or digital chatter dulls the clinician's empathic receptors. Silence is not absence of information, it is bandwidth for resonance.

10.4 Service as Resonance
10.4.1 Expanding the Definition of Healing

Service is the outward expression of coherence. When a chiropractor helps a dog regain mobility or a mare nurse her foal comfortably, that act ripples outward into human emotional fields and even into community morale. Every coherent barn becomes a beacon of peace within its county.

10.4.2 Ripple Effects in Society

One aligned practice can shift entire social networks. Staff retention improves, clients become more compassionate owners, and interprofessional respect deepens. These are not abstract ideals; they are measurable improvements in tone, communication, and well-being. Resonant service is therefore both healthcare and social care.

Sphere of Influence	Observable Outcome	Metric Example
Animal patient	Calmer behavior, improved HRV	HRV variance ↑30%
Owner / client	Reduced anxiety, trust in profession	Cortisol ↓25%
Clinic staff	Cooperative atmosphere	Employee satisfaction ↑
Community	Positive word-of-mouth, humane culture	Adoption rates ↑

Table 27: Mapping social coherence outcomes of resonant service.

10.4.3 Service as Gratitude in Motion

True resonance is reciprocal. Every adjustment returns the practitioner to humility before life's complexity. Gratitude becomes kinetic; expressed through precision, care, and attention to detail. In that way, every touch is a prayer of thanks.

10.5 The Resonant Team
10.5.1 Building Collective Tone

A clinic's success depends as much on collective nervous-system regulation as on skill. A single anxious staff member can introduce discordant frequencies into the environment. Daily group check-ins and two minutes of shared breathing restore phase alignment among team members.

10.5.2 Interdisciplinary Harmony

Veterinarians, chiropractors, technicians, and owners must learn to operate as an orchestra rather than soloists. Shared goals, transparent data, and mutual respect transform multidisciplinary practice into coherent symphony. Frequency sessions before staff meetings can set the tone for problem-solving and creativity.

10.5.3 Resonant Leadership

Leadership by resonance is not authoritarian; it is gravitational. The leader does not command motion but generates coherence so compelling that others naturally synchronize. The ultimate authority in such an environment is not rank but rhythm.

10.6 Language, Story, and Teaching
10.6.1 Narrative as Bridge

Science persuades the intellect; story opens the heart. The resonant doctor learns to teach through metaphor, turning electromagnetic principles into images the public can feel. Explaining "coherence" as "tuning an orchestra" or "helping the body remember its song" communicates truth without dilution.[1] Story thus becomes pedagogy—carrying frequency through language.

10.6.2 Translating Complexity with Compassion

When discussing PEMF or Qi Coil therapies with owners, avoid the vocabulary of circuitry and instead speak of rhythm, rest, and recovery. Clear, compassionate translation preserves both accuracy and accessibility. The aim is not to impress but to harmonize understanding.

Scientific Term	Accessible Analogue	Emotional Frame
Electromagnetic resonance	"The body's natural rhythm"	Familiarity
Coherence index	"How smoothly energy flows"	Calm
Heart-rate variability	"Balance between rest and activity"	Trust
Phase alignment	"Everything moving together again"	Unity

Table 28: Examples of resonant messaging for clients and communities.

10.6.3 Teaching as Transmission

Every conversation radiates tone. When doctors teach with sincerity, their physiology entrains the listener even before comprehension occurs. The student learns coherence not only from what is said but from how it feels to be near the teacher. This is chiropractic education at its highest frequency.

10.7 The Ethics of Power and Presence
10.7.1 Energetic Authority

To influence another's field is to wield subtle power. Whether via hands or waveform, the practitioner enters sacred territory. Humility, not control, must guide the encounter. Energetic authority arises from integrity—alignment between intention, word, and deed.[2]

10.7.2 Transparency and Consent

Discussing goals, sensations, and safety prior to sessions honors both ethical law and vibrational law. Transparency clarifies the energetic contract: the patient offers trust; the doctor offers coherence. Breach of honesty creates discordant interference.

10.7.3 Compassion as Boundary

Compassion does not mean absorption. The resonant doctor maintains boundaries by remaining grounded in self-coherence, allowing empathy without energetic depletion. Presence becomes protection.

10.8 The Journey of Mastery
10.8.1 Stages of Resonant Development

Stage	Focus	Challenge	Integration Tool
Competence	Technique, safety	Inconsistency	Repetition and feedback
Fluency	Flow, timing	Ego reactivity	Reflection, humility
Resonant Artistry	Intuitive precision	Energy drain	Meditation, gratitude
Coherent Mastery	Effortless empathy	Complacency	Service, continual learning

Table 29 placeholder: stages of professional resonance development.

10.8.2 Resilience Under Stress

True mastery appears when coherence persists amid chaos; an injured horse, an emergency call, a client in grief. The doctor's heartbeat becomes the metronome of calm that steadies the environment. Maintaining rhythm under pressure is the signature of an integrated nervous system.

10.8.3 Lifelong Apprenticeship

Even masters remain students of vibration. Every patient teaches a new tone, every setback refines sensitivity. The path never ends because resonance itself is infinite movement.

10.9 The Legacy of Light
10.9.1 Mentorship as Illumination

Legacy is measured not in wealth or recognition but in coherence transmitted. Each practitioner who mentors another multiplies frequency stability across generations. Written notes, case archives, and oral stories preserve more than information—they preserve vibration.

10.9.2 Community as Continuum

A resonant profession self-organizes like a living neural net. When clinics, schools, and farms maintain open communication, energy circulates rather than stagnates. The community itself becomes an organism of light—each node glowing with mutual reinforcement.

10.9.3 Serving the Future

Stewardship of knowledge carries environmental and ethical responsibility. The doctor who plants trees near barns, reduces electromagnetic pollution, and teaches gentle handling practices extends chiropractic beyond vertebrae to the vertebrae of Earth itself.

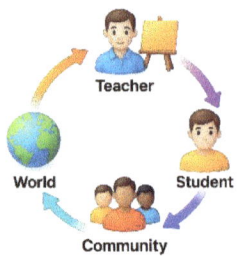

Diagram 14: lineage of illumination.

10.10 Epilogue – The Silence After the Sound

When all the research, waveforms, and adjustments fall away, what remains is silence—the fertile stillness from which all vibration arises. In that silence the resonant doctor listens, breathes, and remembers that healing is not command but communion.

Chiropractic began with a single touch that changed the world's tone. Today, through field technology and awakened consciousness, that tone expands beyond spines to societies, beyond bodies to biospheres. To live the chiropractic way of being is to be the adjustment—a steady pulse of clarity in a noisy world.

May every practitioner who reads these pages walk in coherence, teach through kindness, and leave behind a trail of quiet light.

1. James L. Oschman, Energy Medicine: The Scientific Basis (Edinburgh: Churchill Livingstone, 2016).
2. Rollin McCraty et al., "Heart Rate Variability as a Measure of Coherence," Alternative Therapies in Health and Medicine 7 (2001): 38–48.
3. Ellen Gehrke and Ann Baldwin, "The Horse–Human Heart Connection," Journal of Equine Veterinary Science 32 (2012): 596–603.

Chapter 11: The Living Field — Humanity, Animals, and the Future of Conscious Care

11.1 Introduction – The Awakening Field

Every age of medicine reveals as much about consciousness as it does about biology. The industrial age taught precision and control; the informational age taught systems and feedback. Now, in the coherence age, humanity begins to recognize that healing itself is a shared field phenomenon—that consciousness, magnetism, and compassion are phases of the same continuum.[1]

Animal chiropractic and frequency medicine together model what future healthcare for all beings might look like: participatory, empathic, and ecologically aware. In these disciplines, the boundary between practitioner and patient softens into a relationship of mutual regulation. The resonant doctor adjusts the body; the adjusted body teaches the doctor presence. Each exchange becomes a small act of planetary coherence.

11.2 The Interconnected Web of Life
11.2.1 From Mechanism to Network

The twentieth century conceived the body as machine; the twenty-first sees it as web. Neurons, fascia, and electromagnetic fields intertwine like roots of a forest, communicating through photons and ions rather than gears and wires.[2] When an animal receives a chiropractic adjustment within a coherent frequency field, that vibration travels outward—through herd mates, through caretakers, through the very soil microbes under hoof.

Scale of Life	Resonant Rhythm	Primary Medium	Observable Effect
Cellular	0.1–100 Hz	ionic oscillations	Membrane potential Enzyme regulation
Organismal	1–20 Hz	neuromuscular cycles Electromagnetic coupling	Mobility, HRV
Herd / Social	0.05–0.2 Hz	group entrainment	Behavioral mirroring Collective calm
Ecosystem	Diurnal / geomagnetic cycles	Atmospheric Schumann waves	Biodiversity stability

Table 30: Comparative scales of coherence (cell → ecosystem).

11.2.2 Gaia and Resonance

James Lovelock's Gaia hypothesis proposed Earth as a self-regulating organism.[3] Resonance science supplies the mechanism: electromagnetic coherence unites oceans, atmosphere, flora, fauna, and human thought into one dynamic nervous system.

When veterinarians and chiropractors restore tone within herds, they participate in planetary homeostasis.

11.3 Humanity's Contract with the Animal Kingdom
11.3.1 Reciprocity, Not Dominion

From domestication onward, animals have served humanity; providing food, labor, and companionship. Resonant medicine reframes this relationship as reciprocal stewardship: animals regulate our emotional coherence as surely as we tend their bodies.
Studies show that petting a dog raises human oxytocin while lowering the animal's cortisol—mutual adjustment in biochemical language.[4]

11.3.2 Animals as Co-Teachers

Each species offers a lesson in alignment: horses in grounded grace, dogs in loyal attunement, cattle in patient rhythm. Observing them refines our own tone. In this sense, veterinary chiropractic is not anthropocentric healing but interspecies dialogue.

11.3.3 Ethics of Partnership

To treat an animal is to accept a covenant: respect its autonomy, honor its instinctive wisdom, and act only within the bounds of compassion.
Resonant practice thus becomes both therapy and theology—the sacred act of remembering kinship.

11.4 From Dominance to Dialogue
11.4.1 Two Models of Care

Mechanistic veterinary medicine often operates through control—sedation, confinement, correction. Resonant care invites cooperation, using frequency and gentle adjustment to create safety so that healing unfolds voluntarily.

Paradigm	Mechanistic Approach	Resonant Approach
Practitioner role	Controller / fixer	Partner / facilitator
Animal role	Passive object	Active participant
Communication	Command-response	Feedback-entrainment
Outcome metric	Symptom suppression	Adaptive coherence

Table 31: Contrasts between mechanistic and resonant care models.

11.4.2 Case Reflection

A rescue mare once resistant to touch began relaxing after low-frequency Qi Coil exposure coupled with gentle sacral adjustments. Within weeks, her herd followed her calm lead.

No pharmacology changed, only the frequency of relationship. Dialogue replaced dominance; trust replaced tension.

11.4.3 Cultural Shift

As these examples accumulate, public perception evolves: animals are not machines to be maintained but conscious systems to be harmonized with. Such realization marks civilization's graduation from exploitation to empathy.

11.5 Conscious Technology
11.5.1 Tools with Intention

Technology is neutral until infused with consciousness. Qi Coil, PEMF, and AI-based coherence analytics become extensions of intention when used mindfully—servants of compassion rather than substitutes for it. Before activating a device, the resonant practitioner centers heart rate and breath, ensuring the waveform carries clarity, not chaos.

11.5.2 Designing for Empathy

Future engineering must integrate bioethical algorithms—machines that sense emotional state and modulate output accordingly.
Compassionate design mirrors nature's feedback loops, adjusting intensity to maintain balance rather than domination.

11.5.3 The Moral Engineer

Those who build and operate such devices assume moral responsibility equal to that of physicians. Frequency medicine without ethics risks becoming noise; with ethics, it becomes symphony. The next frontier is therefore not faster computation but purer intention.

11.6 The Planetary Nervous System
11.6.1 Earth as Organism

The magnetic pulses that travel through Earth's crust and atmosphere are the same frequencies that sustain circadian rhythm and cellular communication. In effect, the planet already functions as a nervous system, conducting information through geomagnetic lines of force.[1] Humanity and animals are not passengers within this field—they are neurons in its brain.

11.6.2 Environmental Resonance Indicators

Schumann resonance waves are 7.83 Hz as a fundamental tone that synchronizes human and animal brain waves. Geomagnetic stability waves are between 1–3 Hz optimally and they correlate with lower cardiac stress events. Soil microbial oscillation rates are 0.1–1 Hz and are predictive of crop resilience. A herd HRV coherence mean with a coherence index of greater than 0.8 indicates collective calm and productivity.

11.6.3 Coherence as Ecology

When herds, handlers, and habitat oscillate together, fewer resources are wasted, and biological diversity flourishes. The chiropractor adjusting a dairy cow under a soft magnetic field indirectly tunes an acre of soil and a thousand unseen organisms. Thus, animal chiropractic becomes a quiet form of climate action.

11.7 The Medicine of the Future
11.7.1 Predictive and Personalized Resonance

The next generation of coherence platforms will integrate wearable sensors, genome-based frequency mapping, and AI pattern recognition. Each animal's vibrational "signature" will guide individualized adjustment schedules and Qi Coil programs, transforming preventive care into continuous tuning rather than episodic repair.

11.7.2 Participatory Healing

Owners, trainers, and veterinarians will share dashboards displaying HRV trends and environmental coherence. Healing becomes participatory: a herd's well-being visible in real time. Every contributor, human or machine, forms part of a learning network devoted to balance.

11.7.3 Integration with Emerging Sciences

Epigenetics demonstrates that environment and emotion rewrite DNA expression; quantum computing models coherence mathematically. As these disciplines merge, chiropractic's philosophy of Innate Intelligence will be re-articulated in the language of informational physics; ancient wisdom rendered measurable.

11.8 The Moral Biology of Light
11.8.1 Photonic Communication

Emotional State	Dominant Wavelength (nm)	Observed Pattern
Fear / Anxiety	630 -640	Fragmented spikes
Neutral Rest	560 - 580	Stable low amplitude
Compassion / Joy	500 - 520	Coherent sinusoid
Meditative Stillness	480 - 490	Sustained luminescence

Table 32 placeholder: photonic and emotional frequency correlations.

Every living cell emits ultra-weak photons that synchronize metabolic timing.[2] These biophotons appear to carry emotional and cognitive information as well. Under stress, emission becomes chaotic; under gratitude, it becomes rhythmic. Light is thus both messenger and mirror of moral state.

11.8.2 Ethical Radiance

Because emotion alters photon emission, the moral life of the practitioner becomes part of clinical hygiene. Kindness literally brightens the room. The "moral biology of light" affirms that goodness is not abstraction but wavelength.

11.8.3 Light as Sacrament

When Qi Coil fields or manual adjustments restore order, they do so by re-aligning light within matter. In that instant, physics and prayer are indistinguishable.

11.9 The Great Synthesis

11.9.1 Science, Art, Spirit

Resonance is the meeting point of knowledge, creativity, and reverence. Science supplies measurement; art, the language of feeling; spirit, the motive to serve. Together they form a trinity of coherence.

11.9.2 Animal Chiropractic as Prototype

Among healing professions, animal chiropractic uniquely integrates structure, motion, and consciousness across species. It stands as a working model for planetary medicine—demonstrating that care need not dominate to be effective, nor mystify to be meaningful.

11.9.3 Holism Reimagined

The future healer will be evaluated not by the number of patients served but by the coherence generated. Success becomes measurable in harmony.

11.10 Closing Invocation – The Field Remembers

When the hands of a chiropractor rest upon an animal's spine, the universe takes a breath. All of history, the magnets of D. D. Palmer, the frequencies of Tesla, the compassion of every healer who ever lived; converges in that moment of alignment. The field remembers.

The resonance built through generations does not end with this book; it continues in every practitioner who chooses intention over impulse, service over status, coherence over chaos.

In the quiet that follows each adjustment, one can hear the oldest sound in existence: the hum of life recognizing itself. May that hum guide your work, your relationships, and your stewardship of this luminous planet. May every thought and action you send into the world travel as clear tone, healing the unseen distances between all living things.

1. Mae-Wan Ho, The Rainbow and the Worm: The Physics of Organisms, 3rd ed. (Singapore: World Scientific, 2008).
2. Fritz-Albert Popp and Konrad Regel, "Biophoton Emission in the Brain," Integrative Physiological and Behavioral Science 29 (1994): 383–393.
3. James L. Oschman, Energy Medicine: The Scientific Basis (Edinburgh: Churchill Livingstone, 2016).

Chapter 12: The Continuum of Light
Practice, Presence, and the Infinite Field

12.1 Introduction – Beyond the Last Page

Books end; fields do not. Every paragraph written before this one has been a pulse within a single, ongoing vibration: life learning to know itself through coherence. The resonant doctor's journey therefore continues after the final sentence, as practice, breath, and relationship.

This twelfth chapter is not a conclusion but a continuum—an invitation to live research. Each animal adjusted, each waveform calibrated, each act of compassion contributes to the grand experiment of creation refining its tone. Knowledge becomes participation. To live beyond the last page means to view every moment as data and every heartbeat as peer-review.

12.2 The Practitioner as Living Laboratory
    12.2.1 The Body as Instrument

The resonant chiropractor's own physiology is laboratory, instrument, and subject. Heart-rate variability, sleep patterns, and mood provide real-time feedback about personal coherence.[1] By observing their own fluctuations with the same curiosity reserved for patients, practitioners maintain scientific humility and spiritual discipline simultaneously.

    12.2.2 Integrating Empirical and Experiential Logs

Traditional research values numbers; wisdom values narrative. The new paradigm merges both. A simple daily log can include HRV readings, perceived energy level, emotional tone, and notable patient responses. Over weeks, correlations emerge between practitioner state and clinical outcomes.

Such hybrid documentation honors both the measurable and the mysterious—the twin languages of chiropractic science.

12.3 Communities of Resonance
    12.3.1 From Solo Practice to Collective Field

Coherence amplifies when shared. Small circles of practitioners can meditate together, compare case data, and create Resonant Guilds; micro-communities dedicated to mutual calibration. When one member stabilizes tone, all benefit through empathic resonance.[2]

12.3.2 Global Networks of Coherence

Digital platforms now allow heart-rate and electromagnetic data to sync across continents. A vet adjusting horses in Texas can participate in the same coherence session as a chiropractor treating dairy cows in Finland. Distance becomes a variable, not a barrier.

12.3.3 Peer Accountability as Energetic Hygiene

Community prevents dogma or isolation. Just as instruments in an orchestra tune to one another, practitioners tune through collegial dialogue, maintaining ethical clarity and technical precision.

12.4 Resonance in Education and Governance
12.4.1 Teaching Through Tone

Educational reform will eventually recognize coherence as learning outcome. Students who regulate their physiology before exams not only recall more information but transmit calm into clinical settings. The how of learning becomes as vital as the what.

12.4.2 Policy Rooted in Empathy

Licensing boards and continuing-education committees can measure professional tone using HRV averages or peer-evaluated coherence indices, complementing existing metrics of competency. Ethical regulation thereby evolves from punitive oversight to supportive resonance.

12.4.3 Institutional Tone

An organization, like a body, has HRV. Policies written in fear constrict; those written in trust expand. Coherence analytics could one day inform meeting protocols, building design, and curriculum pacing—making education itself a living organism.

12.5 The Role of the Artist and Storyteller
12.5.1 Art as Frequency Translation

The artist renders invisible vibration visible. Film, sculpture, and sound can illustrate coherence for audiences resistant to technical jargon. Veterinary schools might one day use animated frequency spectrums to teach emotion–physiology coupling.[3]

12.5.2 Color and Tone Pedagogy

Artists intuitively grasp resonance: cool hues calm, warm hues activate. Linking frequency sets to color wheels helps practitioners feel the medicine they deliver. For instance, the 7.8

Hz "Calm Earth" tone may correspond visually to deep indigo; 14 Hz "Focus" to vibrant gold.

12.5.3 Story as Field Maintenance

Narratives keep energy flowing through time. When practitioners share case stories publicly, they maintain vibrational continuity across generations. The telling itself is adjustment—a recalibration of collective memory toward hope.

12.6 The Silence Between Frequencies
12.6.1 The Pause as Practice

Between every wave lies stillness—the gap that allows rhythm to exist. In a world obsessed with motion and metrics, the resonant doctor must defend that gap. Silence is not absence; it is the resonant medium through which meaning travels.[1]

A short pause before beginning a session allows the practitioner's nervous system to entrain downward from sympathetic anticipation into parasympathetic receptivity. This "micro-sabbath" returns accuracy to touch and authenticity to communication.

12.6.2 Integrative Stillness

Just as muscles require recovery after exertion, consciousness requires assimilation after insight. Scheduling intentional silence in professional life ensures that knowledge crystallizes into wisdom rather than fatigue. In that stillness, intuition matures into reliable data.

12.7 The Quantum Nature of Compassion
12.7.1 Entanglement as Metaphor for Love

Quantum physics describes particles separated by distance yet instantly linked through entanglement. Compassion functions similarly: an empathic act in one heart alters the coherence of another thousands of miles away.[2] The chiropractor's focused kindness in a barn or kennel subtly informs the entire professional field.

12.7.2 Scientific Correlates

Laboratory studies on intention-imprinted water and remote heart-to-heart coherence suggest that consciousness modulates electromagnetic patterns independent of physical proximity.[3] These findings imply that compassion is not sentiment but biophysics—an energetic bridge uniting mind and matter.

12.7.3 Ethical Implications

If compassion truly reorganizes matter, indifference becomes a form of entropy. Every thought carries moral resonance. The quantum nature of love demands disciplined awareness: to maintain coherence even when unseen.

12.8 The Field of the Future
12.8.1 Cross-Species Hospitals

Imagine a healing campus where veterinarians, chiropractors, agronomists, and engineers collaborate under one resonant roof. Horses recover beside human athletes, both monitored by frequency sensors tuned to individual harmonic profiles. Treatment plans become compositions; adjustments, light, and sound orchestrated in real time.

12.8.2 Integration with Planetary Analytics

Satellite-linked magnetometers could one day correlate herd coherence with geomagnetic data, predicting stress events before disease manifests. Veterinary resonance labs would double as environmental observatories, merging medicine and climatology.

12.8.3 The Role of the Practitioner

Even in a technologically advanced era, the human nervous system remains the most sophisticated detector and transmitter of resonance. Machines may measure tone; only consciousness can choose harmony.

12.9 The Infinite Feedback Loop
12.9.1 Evolution as Adjustment

The universe perpetually self-corrects—stars oscillate, ecosystems rebalance, cells repair. Chiropractic mirrors this cosmic rhythm: detect distortion, apply gentle correction, allow adaptation. Humanity's role is to cooperate with, not control, that process.

12.9.2 Matter, Energy, and Consciousness

Modern physics dissolves boundaries between these domains: matter is condensed energy; energy is organized consciousness. Each informs the other in infinite recursion. The doctor's adjustment alters posture; posture alters perception; perception alters world.

12.9.3 Participating in the Loop

Every practitioner's coherence contributes to the universe's self-healing. The more awareness flows through this loop, the smoother evolution proceeds. To live resonantly is to assist creation in adjusting itself.

12.10 Benediction – The Light We Share

There is a moment, after a perfect adjustment or a session of deep frequency stillness, when breath suspends and time dilates. In that instant, one feels the world exhale. That is the sound of unity remembered.

This light; your light; is the universe recognizing itself in service. Every act of care, every note of compassion, is an echo of creation refining its music. Carry that melody into barns, clinics, classrooms, and conversations. Let your life be the waveform by which others find their tone.

When all instruments play in coherence, the field becomes luminous beyond measure, and healing, at last, becomes another name for love.

1. James L. Oschman, Energy Medicine: The Scientific Basis (Edinburgh: Churchill Livingstone, 2016).
2. Dean Radin, Entangled Minds: Extrasensory Experiences in a Quantum Reality (New York: Simon & Schuster, 2006).
3. Rollin McCraty et al., "Coherence: Bridging Personal, Social, and Global Health," Frontiers in Public Health 9 (2021): 1–15.

Chapter 13: Applied Resonance
Tools, Protocols, and Integration Models

13.1 Introduction – From Principle to Procedure

Philosophy becomes medicine only when it learns to walk. The previous chapters have explored why coherence matters; this chapter explains how to bring it to life in barns, kennels, and clinics. The bridge from theory to practice is rhythm; structured repetition that transforms insight into habit.

Applied resonance demands systems as elegant as the physics that inspire it. Clear models, predictable schedules, and intentional integration allow chiropractic and frequency therapies to operate with both rigor and grace. Each tool; Qi Coil, PEMF, laser, or sound; becomes a verse within the same song.

13.2 The Five-Step Integration Model for Practitioners

The 5-Step Resonant Integration Model provides a repeatable framework aligning mechanical, electromagnetic, and emotional elements of care. It is less a checklist than a choreography of coherence.

In step one the focus is on centering to allow the practitioner to establish coherence and establish rhythmic HRV and breath alignment. This can be accomplished with 3-minutes of diaphragmatic breathing with 7.8 Hz Earth-tone field playing.

Step two is the assessment of the patient with a structural and energetic scan allowing the identification of subluxations and field asymmetries. This can be done with palpation and completion of the "Show Me Animal Chiropractic" assessments.

Step three is the adjustment and restoration of mechanical and field correction of subluxation by delivering a specific chiropractic adjustment while entraining nervous system. The manual thrust can be given while playing the Qi Coil at 10–12 Hz.

Step four is the integration phase to allow for post-adjustment stabilization. This reinforces neurological pattern and cellular metabolism. 3–5 min PEMF at 5 Hz + red laser (650 nm) will accomplish very efficiently.

Step five is the reflection and documentation phase which allows for feedback from the patient and for any adaptation for the next time. The practitioner records outcomes and refine future care. "Show Me Animal Chiropractic" results are noted along with any HRV, and owner reports of changes.

Each phase honors a principle of chiropractic philosophy:
    Centering echoes the Law of Tone.
    Assessment reflects Specificity.
    Adjustment expresses Intelligence through action.
    Integration respects Time.

Reflection embodies Innate's communication back to Source.

13.3 Example Daily Schedules

Rhythm sustains coherence; scheduling transforms intuition into reliability. The following models illustrate balanced energy management for both practitioner and patient.

13.3.1 Clinic Setting (Small Animal Practice)

Morning Cycle

8:00 – 8:15 a.m.   Team centering: group breathing and HRV check.
8:15 – 12:00 p.m.   Patient sessions using 7–10 Hz Qi Coil pre-field, followed by adjustment and short PEMF integration.
12:00 – 1:00 p.m.   Quiet lunch with 5 Hz recovery frequency playing softly in background.

Afternoon Cycle

1:00 – 4:30 p.m.   Patient sessions using 7–10 Hz Qi Coil pre-field, followed by adjustment and short PEMF integration
4:30 – 5:00 p.m.   Team debrief: review HRV trends, client feedback, and clinic field tone.

This rhythm yields roughly 50 patients per day while maintaining energetic stability. The team ensures that each patient receives the correct amount of and appropriate frequency of PEMF therapy allowing the doctor to focus their attention on the adjustment and removal of vertebral subluxations.

13.3.2 Farm or Field Setting (Large Animal Practice)

Morning Preparation

Check ambient EM field (avoid high-voltage lines).
Ground equipment; set Qi Coil dual units to 5–8 Hz baseline.

Working Block

For individual animals 6 to 10 animals per hour depending on species: pre-field exposure 2 min, adjustment, then post-field PEMF for 10 min. Using a coil that can influence 3,000 square feet allows the PEMF therapy to be administered to multiple animals at the same time.

For herds of animals the PEMF therapy remains the same, at least 2 minutes prior to the adjustment and 10 minutes after the adjustment. The adjustment is aimed at improving resonance and organization of the animal (Principle 32. Coordination. Harmonious action of all parts of an organism in fulfilling their purposes) and the herd. Paying attention to specific areas of the spine that cause issues with this principle will vary from species to species but also purpose of the flock or herd the doctor is working with. Breeding or meat production are different purposes.

Rotate to next animal while first completes integration phase.

Afternoon Group Coherence

20-min herd relaxation session with low-frequency broadcast (4–6 Hz).

Environmental monitoring and documentation of behavioral changes (calmness, social interaction).

Evening Recovery

Practitioner self-care: 5-min alpha frequency meditation, gentle stretching, hydration, HRV review.

13.4 Blending Qi Coil with PEMF, Laser, and Sound Therapy
    13.4.1 Complementary Modalities

Each technology engages a different level of biologic resonance. When combined with chiropractic adjustment, they operate like harmonics in a chord: distinct, yet unified by intent.

Modality	Primary Mechanism	Resonant Synergy	Application Tip
Qi Coil System	Tunable pulsed electromagnetic field (PEMF)	Nervous-system entrainment and emotional coherence	5–15 Hz during or immediately after adjustment
PEMF Mat or Loop	Deep-tissue microcirculation and ion mobilization	Enhances metabolic recovery post-adjustment	Alternate days or rotate with Qi Coil for depth variance
Cold Laser (LLLT)	Photonic stimulation of mitochondria at 660–850 nm	Increases ATP and supports tissue oxygenation	Sweep over adjusted region 2–3 min post-session
Sound Therapy / 432 Hz Tones	Acoustic pressure wave entrainment through air	Reinforces parasympathetic tone and emotional ease	Play ambiently at ≤ 60 dB during sessions

Table 33: Comparison of multimodal resonance therapies.

13.4.2 Layered Application

Prepare: Qi Coil 5 Hz baseline for 2 minutes while the animal settles.

Adjust: Manual correction with 10–12 Hz entrainment.

Stabilize: Cold laser (660 nm) 2–3 minutes on adjusted segments.

Reinforce: PEMF 5 Hz for 5 minutes while playing 432 Hz ambient tone.

This "stacked resonance" protocol addresses structure (mechanics), energy (field), and emotion (affect) simultaneously.

13.4.3 Safety and Sequencing

Avoid overlap of high-amplitude PEMF and laser directly over pacemaker implants.

Maintain grounding of metal stalls and equipment.

Always re-center personal coherence before re-activating the next device cycle.

13.5 Patient and Client Education & Compliance Tools

13.5.1 Communicating the Why

Owners and handlers embrace programs they understand. Translate technical concepts into everyday imagery:

"Your animal's nervous system is like an orchestra. The adjustment tunes each instrument; the Qi Coil keeps the music in tune between visits."

Visual proof strengthens trust: "Show Me Animal Chiropractic" differences. HRV graphs, before-and-after thermographic images, or slow-motion videos of improved gait turn the invisible into visible science.

13.5.2 Home and Barn Compliance Aids

After-care Frequency cards reinforce home use protocols helping maintain resonant frequencies between visits. "5 Hz Calm Set – twice daily for 5 min".
QR code video links that educate the owner on why and how to help both themselves and their animals. These may be embedded in follow-up emails. "Owner breathing or coherence training".
Text Reminders / App Notifications to encourage daily practice and data logging of their observations reinforcing the importance of doing the home work. "Today's calm session due at 6 p.m."

Help the owner understand that the "Owner Observation Log" where they can track behavioral and physiologic changes, issues like changes in appetite, energy, mobility, and demeanor by assigning a team member to look at and make copies of if necessary to include in patient records.

13.5.3 Outcome Tracking and Dialogue

During re-evaluations, review owner logs alongside objective data ("Show Me Animal Chiropractic" results, HRV, gait video). Co-interpretation empowers clients as partners in care. Education thus becomes co-creation, a shared act of keeping the field coherent.

13.6 Conclusion – The Practice of Harmony

Integration is the final adjustment. When routine meets reverence, systems become ceremony. Whether in a city clinic or a rural barn, these protocols anchor coherence in the ordinary rhythm of workdays. Schedules, checklists, and technologies do not diminish vitalism, they manifest it. They turn philosophy into habit, habit into culture, and culture into legacy.

Each office, farm, or mobile practice that adopts the five-step model, harmonic scheduling, and education tools becomes a node of global resonance, a place where the laws of tone govern both healing and daily life.

1. C. Andrew Bassett et al., "Effects of Pulsing Electromagnetic Fields on Bone Repair," Journal of Bone and Joint Surgery 58-A (1976): 993–1003.
2. James L. Oschman, Energy Medicine: The Scientific Basis (Edinburgh: Churchill Livingstone, 2016).
3. Rollin McCraty et al., "Coherence: Bridging Personal, Social, and Global Health," Frontiers in Public Health 9 (2021): 1–15.

Chapter 14 Living in Coherence — The Practitioner as the Field

14.1 Introduction – The Doctor as Environment

Every practitioner is a living ecosystem. The electromagnetic signature of one's own heart, breath, and intention quietly conditions the physiology of the beings one touches. Whether human, horse, or hound, each patient responds not merely to the technique applied but to the frequency state of the hands that deliver it. The doctor is part of the intervention.

To live and practice in coherence is therefore both scientific discipline and moral vocation. It requires that one's internal terrain — hydration, diet, circadian rhythm, thought — become as carefully tended as any clinic or barn. Energy hygiene is professional hygiene.

Chiropractic's earliest philosophy recognized that healing arises when interference is removed from life's expression. The modern extension of that insight is that the practitioner's incoherence can itself be a subtle interference. Hence, self-care is not indulgence; it is ethical necessity.

14.2 Practitioner Self-Care and Energy Hygiene

14.2.1 Physical Coherence

Body chemistry dictates field clarity. Regular movement, consistent hydration, and full-spectrum daylight recalibrate circadian oscillators that anchor electromagnetic rhythm. Chronic dehydration or sleep disruption increases oxidative noise, lowering HRV and diminishing empathic precision.[1] A coherent practice day therefore begins the night before, with rest and mineral balance.

14.2.2 Emotional and Cognitive Boundaries

Empathy without boundaries becomes absorption. Between sessions, five deliberate breaths or a brief visualization of light returning to the heart acts as an energetic "hand-washing." Gratitude journaling before leaving the office reframes fatigue as fulfillment, transmuting sympathetic drive into parasympathetic repair.

14.2.3 Energetic Routine

It is important to remember to take care of yourself and your team first. No one can help others heal if they are sick themselves. It is difficult to raise the vibration level of those around you if your vibration level is at a low level. Each morning should start with a personal check in, with at least a mid-day recheck before winding down every evening.

Practitioners should schedule time away from patients and time to indulge in things that they enjoy. George I. Bernard, D.C. stated that to be the best in any field you must love what you do. Regularly prioritizing self-care prevents burnout, strengthens relationships, and improves your ability to handle life's challenges with greater resilience.

Self-care allows you to bring a better you to the patient every time. Taking time improves the mental and emotional health of the individual by:
1) Reduces stress and anxiety: Me-time provides a necessary break to relax and unwind, which can significantly lower stress and anxiety levels and improve your mood.
2) Boosts emotional regulation: Solitude offers a chance to observe and regulate your emotions, leading to greater emotional balance and a sense of peace.
3) Increases self-awareness: Alone time helps you listen to your thoughts and feelings without distraction, promoting self-reflection and a deeper understanding of yourself.

Self-care provides benefits for physical health by:
1) Improves sleep: Taking time to rest and recharge can lead to better sleep and more energy.
2) Boosts energy levels: Regular self-care practices can increase your energy and help you manage the demands of daily life.
3) Supports overall physical health. Managing stress and caring for your mental well-being, also lowers your risk of illness.

Self-care helps your productivity and creativity by:
1) When your mind is relaxed and free from social pressures, you can explore your interests, plan for the future, and discover creative solutions to problems.
2) Taking regular breaks and engaging in self-care activities can help you return to tasks refreshed, leading to increased focus and efficiency.

Taking care of yourself will benefit your relationships.
1) It will improve existing relationships: By taking care of your own needs, you can strengthen your relationships with family and friends and become more present and compassionate.
2) Fosters independence: Spending time alone can build confidence in your ability to be independent, act on your own, and find enjoyment by yourself.

14.2.4 Environmental Hygiene

Clean field equals clean mind. Ground electrical equipment, reduce fluorescent flicker, and use 432 Hz ambient tones in treatment rooms. Even the layout of furniture affects magnetic flow, clutter breeds noise. Simplicity is resonance embodied.

14.3 Developing Intuitive Resonance in Healing Work
    14.3.1 Intuition as Learned Resonance

Intuition is not mysticism but refined pattern recognition within the sensory field. The nervous system of a seasoned practitioner continuously samples micro-movements, temperature gradients, and subtle rhythmic shifts, translating them into felt impressions. This somatic literacy arises from exposure, humility, and trust in perception.

14.3.2 Exercises for Refinement

Breath Mirroring: Before contact, observe the animal's respiratory cadence and silently match it until both settle into one rhythm.

Pulse Alignment: At rest position, feel for arterial rhythm; wait until practitioner's heartbeat entrains.

Still-point Listening: Maintain gentle contact at atlas or sacrum; when internal chatter stops and the tissue softens spontaneously, record duration and sensory cues.

Post-Session Reflection: Immediately note any imagery or temperature changes perceived; over months, pattern recognition sharpens.

These practices cultivate what early chiropractors called listening through the hands—a communion that joins neurophysiology and empathy.

14.3.3 Scientific Correlates

Heart–brain research shows measurable synchronization of heart-rate variability between people and animals during empathic interaction.[2] Coherence is contagious; presence is physics. As practitioners develop intuitive resonance, they become instruments tuned for perception as much as for adjustment.

14.4 Teaching Patients and Clients the Language of Energy
14.4.1 Translating Resonance into Everyday Speech

The art of explanation is itself a frequency bridge. When the practitioner uses imagery drawn from familiar experience, abstract physics becomes relatable empathy. Energy need not be mystified to be meaningful. For instance:

"Your animal's body is like a communication network. Each nerve signal is a message. When one joint becomes jammed, it's like static on the line. The adjustment clears that static, and frequency therapies keep the message clear."

In a single sentence, quantum coherence, mechanoreception, and chiropractic philosophy converge into language any owner can feel.

Analogy	Scientific Correlate	Teaching Context
"Tuning an instrument"	Neurological phase synchronization	Performance animals
"Resetting a circuit breaker"	Spinal reflex modulation	Acute injury
"Clearing static on a radio"	Improved afferent signal-to-noise ratio	Companion animals
"Finding the rhythm again"	HRV coherence	Geriatric or anxious cases

Table 2 placeholder: analogies linking everyday imagery with physiological mechanisms.

14.4.2 Experiential Learning

Clients often learn more from sensation than from explanation. Invite them to breathe slowly with their animal as the Qi Coil hums softly. When both heart rhythms settle into visible coherence on a monitor, the concept ceases to be theory; it becomes shared experience.

14.4.3 Empowering Self-Observation

Educated clients become co-regulators rather than passive recipients. Teach them to notice posture, breath, and demeanor as barometers of tone. In doing so, you awaken their innate diagnostic faculty—an extension of Innate Intelligence into daily stewardship.

14.5 The Chiropractic Adjustment as Mechanical and Vibrational Act
14.5.1 The Dual Nature of the Adjustment

An adjustment is both structure and song. Mechanically, it restores joint motion and resets proprioceptive feedback. Energetically, it delivers a coherent impulse, an acoustic shock wave through bone and fascia; that re-synchronizes neural oscillators.[1] The audible cavitation, once seen merely as gas release, can be understood as an acoustic marker of phase shift: matter briefly reorganizing around a new equilibrium.

14.5.2 Mechanotransduction and Electromagnetic Coupling

Cells translate mechanical force into bioelectric signals via stretch-activated ion channels and piezoelectric matrices. When a thrust is delivered with precision and intent, the local crystalline lattice of connective tissue converts pressure into current—a flash of coherent light at the nanoscale.[2] Thus, every adjustment is also photonic communication.

14.5.3 The Adjustment as Dialogue

True correction is conversation, not command. The practitioner listens, applies measured input, and waits for tissue reply. This bidirectional exchange; force and feedback, tone and counter-tone; is the essence of vibrational medicine within chiropractic's mechanical act.

14.6 Conclusion – Living the Adjustment

Living in coherence means carrying the state of adjustment beyond the table.
The same rhythm that guides the thrust should guide speech, rest, and relationship.
Each breath becomes an alignment, each interaction, a micro-adjustment to the world's tone.

When practitioner and patient, human and animal, touch within shared resonance, the boundaries between anatomy and empathy blur. At that moment, chiropractic fulfills its oldest promise: to remind life how to speak fluently with itself.

The self-caring, intuitive, teaching, and adjusting doctor is not separate from the field—they are the field. To live coherently is to embody the principle that healing is not something we perform; it is something we become.

1. Joshua N. Hong et al., "Mechanotransduction in Bone and Soft Tissue," Frontiers in Bioengineering and Biotechnology 12 (2023): 1–12.
2. James L. Oschman, Energy Medicine: The Scientific Basis (Edinburgh: Churchill Livingstone, 2016).

Appendix D Glossary of Vibrational Medicine Terms

Preface: Using This Glossary in Practice and Education

This glossary serves as both a reference guide and a teaching tool for clinicians, veterinary students, and chiropractic educators who are exploring the interface between biomechanics and bioenergetics. Each entry is concise but context-rich, bridging conventional anatomy and the language of vibrational medicine. Use glossary entries in client education materials to explain complex ideas with precise yet accessible language. Encourage multidisciplinary dialogue—veterinary, chiropractic, and physics alike—through shared vocabulary. The glossary reflects the language of coherence: a lexicon where physics meets physiology and philosophy informs practice.

A

Amplitude — The maximum displacement of a wave from its baseline; in frequency therapy, amplitude correlates with field intensity (measured in millitesla, mT).
Autonomic Coherence — A physiologic state in which sympathetic and parasympathetic branches of the nervous system oscillate in harmonic rhythm, often measurable through heart-rate variability (HRV).

B

Bioresonance — Interaction between biologic tissues and externally applied frequencies intended to restore energetic balance.
Biophoton — Ultra-weak light emitted by cells as part of metabolic signaling, first measured by Fritz-Albert Popp in the 1970s.
Biofield — The aggregate electromagnetic and informational field produced by living systems.

C

Coherence — Orderly, synchronized oscillation among multiple systems (e.g., heart, brain, fascia). In practice, coherence is both a measurable biophysical condition and a subjective sense of ease or flow.
Constructive Interference — When two waves of similar frequency align in phase, increasing total amplitude; central to harmonic stacking in PEMF and Qi Coil applications.
Cymatics — The visual study of sound and vibration patterns in matter (e.g., sand or water); demonstrates how frequency organizes form.

D

Detoxification Frequencies — Low-amplitude electromagnetic signals (typically 0.5–4 Hz) believed to support lymphatic and cellular waste removal.

Damping — Reduction of oscillation amplitude over time due to resistance; in tissue, damping represents the natural absorption of mechanical or electromagnetic energy.

E

Electromagnetic Induction — The process by which a changing magnetic field generates an electric current; principle underlying PEMF and Qi Coil design.
Entrapment / Entrainment — Tendency of one oscillating system to synchronize with another of similar frequency; e.g., heart–brain or practitioner–patient coherence.

F

Frequency — Number of oscillations per second, measured in hertz (Hz). Biological systems respond to specific frequency "windows."
Fascia — Continuous connective-tissue network that conducts both mechanical tension and subtle bioelectric signals.
Field Strength — Magnetic flux density within the treatment zone, typically expressed in microtesla (µT) or millitesla (mT).

G

Grounding — Establishing electrical connection between the body or device and the Earth to stabilize charge and reduce electromagnetic noise.

H

Harmonic Stacking — Overlay of multiple related frequencies (fundamental F, overtones 2F–4F) to broaden physiologic resonance.
Heart-Rate Variability (HRV) — Variation in time between heartbeats; higher HRV indicates balanced autonomic function and greater adaptability.

I

Innate Intelligence — Chiropractic term describing the inherent organizing principle of living matter; analogous to systemic coherence in physics.
Interference Pattern — Composite waveform resulting when two or more fields intersect; can be constructive or destructive.

M

Mechanotransduction — Conversion of mechanical force into cellular biochemical or electrical signals; key link between chiropractic adjustment and bioelectric response.
Mitochondrial Resonance — Hypothesized alignment of external frequency with mitochondrial membrane potential (~0.1 V) to enhance ATP production.

N

Neuromagnetic Realignment — Integrative concept describing simultaneous mechanical and electromagnetic correction during adjustment.

Noise (Energetic) — Random, non-coherent vibration that obscures or disrupts biologic signaling.

P

PEMF (Pulsed Electromagnetic Field) — Therapeutic use of time-varying magnetic fields to influence cellular and nervous-system activity.

Phase Locking — Stable synchronization of oscillations between two systems; basis for entrainment phenomena.

Piezoelectricity — Electric charge generated by mechanical stress in crystalline structures such as collagen and bone.

Q

Qi Coil — Portable toroidal-field frequency-therapy device based on Tesla-coil and scalar-wave principles, controlled via mobile application.

Quantum Coherence — State in which subatomic particles maintain phase relationships across a system; used metaphorically in energy medicine to describe synchronized biological processes.

R

Resonance — Amplification of oscillation when a system is exposed to its natural frequency; central mechanism of vibrational healing.

Rife Frequencies — Discrete frequencies developed by Royal Raymond Rife (1930s) purported to disrupt pathogenic resonance; modern adaptations use safe low-energy analogues.

S

Scalar Field — Hypothetical non-vector energy field without direction but with magnitude; referenced in Tesla-derived and toroidal technologies.

Schumann Resonance — Earth's fundamental electromagnetic standing wave (~7.83 Hz) associated with circadian and autonomic regulation.

Subluxation (Chiropractic) — Functional misalignment causing neurologic interference; viewed here as both structural and vibrational distortion.

T

Toroidal Field — Doughnut-shaped magnetic configuration that circulates energy in closed loops; design geometry of Qi Coil systems.

Tone — Original chiropractic metaphor for life's vibrational harmony; equivalent to coherence at the physiologic and spiritual level.

V

Vibrational Medicine — Therapeutic paradigm using frequency, sound, or electromagnetic energy to restore harmony within living systems.

Vagus Tone — Physiologic indicator of parasympathetic dominance; higher tone corresponds to relaxation and homeostasis.

W

Waveform — Shape of an oscillating signal (sine, square, sawtooth); determines qualitative tissue response.

Water Memory — Controversial hypothesis that liquid water can retain structural imprint of electromagnetic fields; ongoing subject of biophysical study.

Z

Zero-Point Field — Quantum vacuum energy present even at absolute zero; proposed energetic substrate of coherence and consciousness.

1. Oschman, James L. Energy Medicine: The Scientific Basis. Edinburgh: Churchill Livingstone, 2016.
2. McCraty, Rollin, and Mike Atkinson. "Resonant Frequency and Heart-Rate Variability: Applications for Stress Reduction." Frontiers in Public Health 9 (2021): 1–12. https://doi.org/10.3389/fpubh.2021.671010
3. Popp, Fritz-Albert, and L. Regel. "Biophoton Emission in the Brain." Integrative Physiology and Behavioral Science 29 (1994): 383–93.

Appendix B Frequency Reference Charts — Common Sets and Targets

A.1 Overview

The following tables summarize core frequency ranges and harmonic groupings used in Qi Coil and related PEMF applications for chiropractic and veterinary practice. Frequencies are expressed in hertz (Hz) and organized by physiologic or energetic target. All ranges are drawn from published PEMF, Rife-derived, and vibrational-medicine literature, correlated with empirical clinical outcomes in both human and animal contexts. [1]

Practitioners are reminded that response is individual and species-specific; frequencies are best viewed as guidelines for entrainment, not rigid prescriptions.

A.2 General Wellness and Autonomic Balance

Purpose / Effect	Primary Frequency (Hz)	Range (Hz)	Notes / Mechanism
Grounding / Earth coherence	7.83	7.5–8.0	Schumann resonance; synchronizes cortical and cardiac rhythms.
Calm / Parasympathetic tone	5.0	4.5–6.0	Enhances vagal activation and HRV; ideal for pre-adjustment.
Focus / Mental clarity	13.0	12-15	Beta-low range; supports practitioner alertness.
Rest / Sleep initiation	3.5	3-4	Delta entrainment; pair with dim light
Emotional balance / Centering	10.0	9-11	Alpha band harmonization; cross-species calming.

Table A1: General wellness and autonomic balance frequencies.

A.3 Tissue-Specific and Functional Targets

System / Tissue	Primary Frequency	Secondary Harmonics	Suggested Duration	Clinical Notes
Skeletal muscle relaxation	8.2 Hz	16.4, 24.6	10-15 min	Reduces tension pre-adjustment.
Fascia / connective tissue	13.0 Hz	26.0	8-12 min	Improves glide; combine with stretching.
Peripheral nerve regeneration	4.0 Hz	8.0	10 min	Aligns with axonal growth cone resonance.
Cartilage / joint repair	7.0 Hz	14.0	15 min	Stimulates chondrocyte metabolism.
Bone healing / osteogenesis	15.0 Hz	30.0	20 min	Mirrors orthopedic PEMF parameters.
Circulation / microvascular flow	10.5 Hz	21.0	10 min	Nitric-oxide release modulation
Inflammation control	5.8 Hz	11.6	15 min	Down-regulates cytokine expression.

Table A2: Tissue-specific harmonics.

A.4 Emotional and Behavioral Harmonics (Animals)

Behavioral Goal	Primary Frequency	Species Adjustments	Application Context
Pre-performance focus	14.2 Hz	Horse ↑ +0.5 Hz Dog ↓ –0.3 Hz	Use 5 min before event or transport
Anxiety / stall rest calm	5.0 Hz	Horse ↑ +0.2 Hz Dog same	Pair with dim light and soft voice
Post-competition recovery	7.8 Hz	Horse same Dog ↑ +0.5 Hz	Combine with massage or stretching
Bonding / trust building	10.0 Hz	Cross-species	Owner and animal share same field.
Sleep / overnight kennel rest	3.5 Hz	Dog same Cat ↓ –0.2 Hz	Run 20 min cycle on timer.

Table A3: Emotional and behavioral harmonics for companion and performance animals.

A.5 Harmonic Relationships and Stacking Map

Qi Coil programs often layer two to four harmonic tones to create composite fields. Lower frequencies (< 10 Hz) modulate autonomic rhythm; upper harmonics (10–30 Hz) influence tissue metabolism.

A.6 Usage Notes and Precautions

Begin with lower amplitudes and shorter durations; increase gradually as tolerance develops. Animals typically respond faster to 4–10 Hz than to higher ranges. Avoid simultaneous overlapping fields of identical amplitude but dissonant waveform phase. Always re-establish grounding after multi-frequency sessions.

1. James L. Oschman, Energy Medicine: The Scientific Basis (Edinburgh: Churchill Livingstone, 2016).
2. Andrew A. Bassett et al., "Effects of Pulsing Electromagnetic Fields on Bone Repair," Journal of Bone and Joint Surgery 58-A (1976): 993–1003.
3. Rollin McCraty and Mike Atkinson, "Resonant Frequency and Heart Rate Variability: Applications for Stress Reduction," Frontiers in Public Health 9 (2021): 1–12.

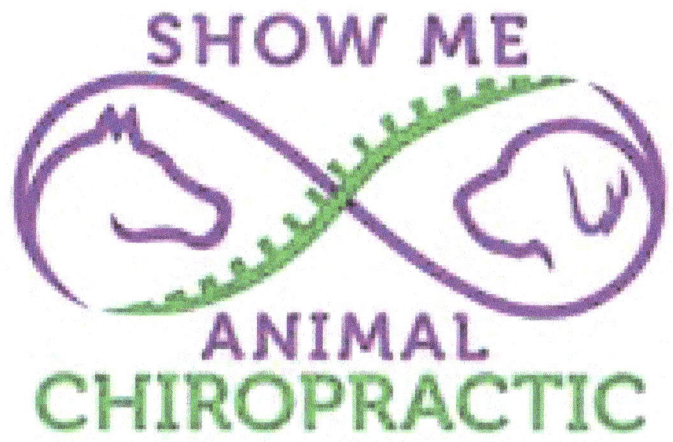

🐾 How to Use Your Show Me Animal Chiropractic Observation Log

🩺 Purpose of This Log

This log helps you track your animal's health, comfort, and response between chiropractic adjustments and Qi Coil sessions. Consistent observations allow your chiropractor to see subtle changes over time — the kind that show the nervous system is adapting and healing. Every note you make helps our team fine-tune care for the best results.

🕐 When to Fill It Out

Daily for the first week after an adjustment or Qi Coil session
Then 2–3 times per week or as recommended
Always note any major change in appetite, behavior, or movement
Bring the completed log to your next appointment

📋 How to Use the Rating Boxes

Each row has checkboxes labeled ☐1–☐5.
Circle or check the number that best describes your observation:

Rating Meanings
- 1 Much worse than usual
- 2 Slightly worse
- 3 Normal / baseline
- 4 Slight improvement
- 5 Marked improvement

You can also write short comments in the Notes column — for example,
"More relaxed after session," or "Eating well but still stiff in right hind."

What to Watch For After a Chiropractic or Qi Coil Session

Improvement is sometimes immediate, but may also unfold over several days as the nervous system resets. Typical signs of positive response include:
- Easier movement and smoother gait
- Calmer demeanor or better focus
- Increased hydration and appetite
- Deeper sleep or more rest
- Improved elimination and digestion

Sometimes, temporary changes (like mild soreness or increased resting) are normal as the body releases stored tension.

Recording Qi Coil Use

If your animal receives Qi Coil sessions at home:
- Record the frequency set or goal used (e.g., "Relaxation," "Pain Relief," "Cellular Recovery")
- Note duration and reaction (calmer, sleepy, more active, etc.)
  - Include this data under "Region Adjusted / Frequency Used" on your log page

This helps the team correlate frequency response with physical changes over time.

Tips for Accurate Observation

Watch at consistent times each day (morning feeding, turnout, or evening rest)
Compare to your animal's normal routine — not to others
Use your senses: sight, touch, sound, and intuition
Stay objective — small improvements matter

Thank You

By filling out these logs, you're part of your animal's healing team. Your observations strengthen the connection between chiropractic care, energy balance, and optimal health.

Show Me Animal Chiropractic — Observation Log
Include this record at your next chiropractic or Qi Coil session.

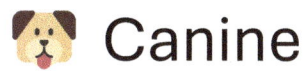 Canine Observation Log

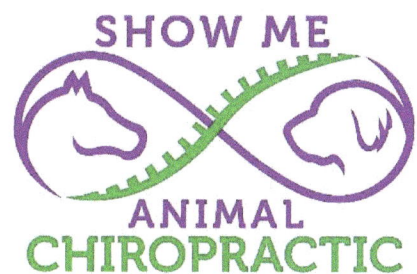

Owner: _____   Dog Name: _____

Breed: _____   Date: _____

1. Daily Wellness

Observation Area	Description / Notes	Rating (1–5)
Appetite / Grain Intake	Ate all feed? Left hay?	☐1 ☐2 ☐3 ☐4 ☐5
Water Consumption	Bucket/tub levels normal?	☐1 ☐2 ☐3 ☐4 ☐5
Activity Level	Playful / Lethargic / Restless?	☐1 ☐2 ☐3 ☐4 ☐5
Mood	Relaxed / Anxious / Aggressive?	☐1 ☐2 ☐3 ☐4 ☐5
Movement	Smooth / Stiff / Limping?	☐1 ☐2 ☐3 ☐4 ☐5

2. Physical Signs

Body Area	Observations
Eyes / Nose	Discharge, squinting, redness, odor, normal
Skin / Coat	Dull, shiny, dryness, itching, hot spots, normal
Gait / Joints	Difficulty jumping or climbing
Digestion	Stool normal / loose / hard
Urination	Frequency, color, control

3. Work & Environment

Factor	Notes
Exercise / Walks	_____
Sleep Quality	_____
Household Stressors	_____
Diet or Treat Changes	_____

4. Chiropractic & Qi Coil Support

Date	Region Adjusted / Frequency Used	Response / Notes

5. Owner Comments

_____

_____

Show Me Animal Chiropractic — Observation Log | Include this record at your next chiropractic or Qi Coil session.

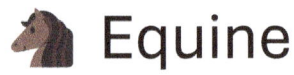 # Equine Observation Log

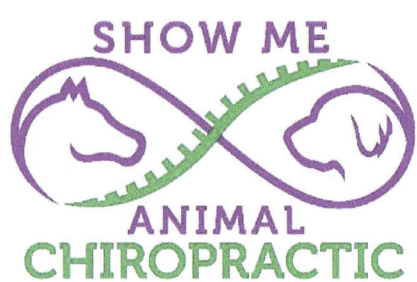

Owner: _____ Horse Name: _____

Breed: _____ Date: _____

1. Daily Wellness

Observation Area	Description / Notes	Rating (1–5)
Appetite / Grain Intake	Ate all feed? Left hay?	☐1 ☐2 ☐3 ☐4 ☐5
Water Consumption	Bucket/tub levels normal?	☐1 ☐2 ☐3 ☐4 ☐5
Manure / Urine	Normal, dry, loose, or reduced?	☐1 ☐2 ☐3 ☐4 ☐5
Attitude / Behavior	Bright / dull / anxious / aggressive	☐1 ☐2 ☐3 ☐4 ☐5
Movement / Gait	Even stride? Shortened step?	☐1 ☐2 ☐3 ☐4 ☐5

2. Physical Signs

Body Area	Observations
Eyes / Nose	Discharge, squinting, rubbing, normal
Skin / Coat	Dull, shiny, sweat patterns, itching, normal
Limbs / Hooves	Heat, swelling, digital pulse, thrush, normal
Back / Neck	Sensitivity, stiffness, asymmetry, normal
Respiratory	Cough, nasal flare, abnormal effort, normal

3. Work & Environment

Factor	Notes
Turnout / Stall Conditions	_____
Workload / Ride Type	_____
Weather / Stress Changes	_____
Feed or Supplement Changes	_____

4. Chiropractic & Qi Coil Support

Date	Region Adjusted / Frequency Used	Response / Notes

5. Owner Comments

_____

_____

Show Me Animal Chiropractic — Observation Log | Include this record at your next chiropractic or Qi Coil session.

🐱 Feline Observation Log

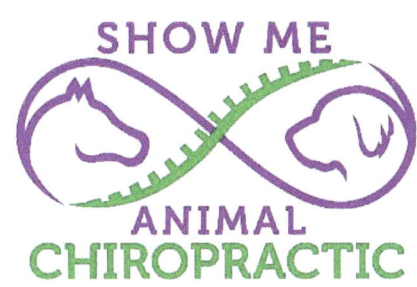

Owner: _____   Cat Name: _____

Breed: _____   Date: _____

1. Daily Wellness

Observation Area	Description / Notes	Rating (1–5)
Appetite	Finished meals? Food avoidance?	☐1 ☐2 ☐3 ☐4 ☐5
Water Intake	Drinking normally?	☐1 ☐2 ☐3 ☐4 ☐5
Litter Box	Normal / Diarrhea / Constipation / None	☐1 ☐2 ☐3 ☐4 ☐5
Grooming	Normal / Excessive / None	☐1 ☐2 ☐3 ☐4 ☐5
Social Behavior	Friendly / Withdrawn / Aggressive	☐1 ☐2 ☐3 ☐4 ☐5

2. Physical Signs

Body Area	Observations
Eyes / Nose	Discharge, squinting
Coat / Skin	Bald spots, dandruff, parasites
Gait / Movement	Jumping easily? Limping?
Breathing	Normal / Rapid / Coughing

3. Work & Environment

Factor	Notes
Indoor / Outdoor Time	_____
Changes in Home Routine	_____
New Pets / People	_____
Diet or Treat Changes	_____

4. Chiropractic & Qi Coil Support

Date	Region Adjusted / Frequency Used	Response / Notes

5. Owner Comments

_____

_____

Show Me Animal Chiropractic — Observation Log | Include this record at your next chiropractic or Qi Coil session.

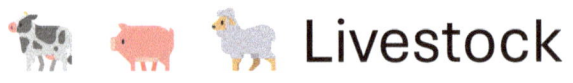 # Livestock Observation Log

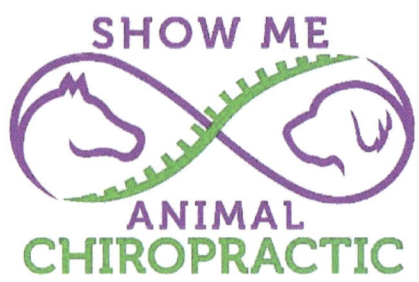

Owner: _____ Animal ID / Tag # / Group: _____

Species: Cattle / Swine / Sheep / Goat / Chicken   Date: _____

1. Feeding & Herd Behavior

Observation	Description	Rating (1–5)
Appetite	Full feed / Off feed / Sorting feed	☐1 ☐2 ☐3 ☐4 ☐5
Water Intake	Normal / Reduced	☐1 ☐2 ☐3 ☐4 ☐5
Social Behavior	Normal / Isolated / Aggressive	☐1 ☐2 ☐3 ☐4 ☐5
Mobility	Normal / Stiff / Lame	☐1 ☐2 ☐3 ☐4 ☐5
Production (milk/weight/eggs)	Stable / Decreasing / Increasing	☐1 ☐2 ☐3 ☐4 ☐5

2. Physical Signs

Category	Notes
Eyes / Nose / Ears	Discharge, drooping, odor
Coat / Skin	Hair loss, scurf, heat spots
Limbs / Hooves	Swelling, tenderness, hoof condition
Udder / Repro	Swelling, discharge, heat, mastitis signs
Feces / Urine	Consistency, color, volume

3. Work & Environment

Factor	Notes
Bedding / Shelter	_____
Weather / Temperature	_____
Feed Change / Source	_____
Herd Dynamics	_____

4. Chiropractic & Qi Coil Support

Date	Region Adjusted / Frequency Used	Response / Notes

5. Owner Comments

_____

_____

Show Me Animal Chiropractic — Observation Log | Include this record at your next chiropractic or Qi Coil session.

Appendix C: QiCoil Frequencies Canine

Treatments (Animal Health Care Professional In House Treatments)

Condition	Treatment
Arthritis	Support Joint Health (Quan), 4698, 570, 146, 1468
Diarrhea	Digestive System Support (Quan), 727.5, 787, 880, 440
Lameness	Support Joint Health (Quan), 1468, 2336, 130, 787
Lack of Appetite	Regenerate (Quan), Cell Metabolism Regenerator (Quan), Get Well Soon, Feel Better (Quan)
Ear Infection	727.5, Colloidal Silver Emulator (Quan), Immune Boost (Quan), 802, 880
Itchy Skin	Psoriasis (Rife), Pruritus (Rife), Dandruff (Rife), Erysipelas (Rife), Immune Boost Max (Quan)
Heart Problems	Heart Restore (Quan), Heart Muscle (Rife), Heart, Cardiac Hypertrophy, Heart (Rife), Heart, Endocarditis (Rife)
Mouth Issues	Dental Infections and Cavitations (Rife), Periodontal Disease (Rife), Gum inflammation (Rife), Tooth Decay (Rife)
Hot Spots	Allergies (Rife), Immune Boost (Rife), Lymphatic System (Rife), Toxin Elimination (Rife), Immune Boost Max (Quan)
Paralyzed Dog	Locomotor Ataxia, Muscle Failure (Rife), Paralysis (Rife), Ataxia of Muscle (Rife), Inflammation (Rife), Support Joint Health (Quan)
Urinary Tract Infections	727.5, 802, Immune Boost Max (Quan), 146, 4698

Appendix E: QiCoil Protocols for Canine Extended Home Use

...er Therapies for at home use by owners

Condition	Protocols
...itis	Support Joint Health (Quan), Arthritis – General (Rife), Joints (Inflamed) (Rife), Osteoarthritis (Rife), 4698, 802, 570, 146, 1468, Nerves, Inflammation (Rife)
...hea	Support Healthy Colon and Bowel (Quan), Immune Boost Max (Quan), 584, Digestive System Support (Quan), 727.5, 787, 880, 440
...eness	Support Joint Health (Quan), Whiplash (Rife), Locomotor Ataxia, Muscle Failu... (Rife), Paralysis (Rife), 2336, 1468, 2336, 130, 787, Muscle Stiffness (Rife), Mu... Repair (Rife),
...of Appetite	Liver Tonic (Quan), Qi Energy Boost (Quan), Inflammation (Rife), Appetite (Lo... (Quan), Appetite, Lack of (Rife)
...Skin	Immune Boost Max (Quan), Skin Restore and Rejuvenate (Quan), Psoriasis (R... Pruritus (Rife) Dandruff (Rife), Erysipelas (Rife), 292,
...h Issues	Dental Infections and Cavitations (Rife), Periodontal Disease (Rife), Gums inflammation (Rife), Tooth Decay (Rife), Bad Teeth (Rife), Immune Boost Max... 146, 4698
...t Problems	Heart Restore (Quan), Heart Muscle (Rife), Heart, Cardiac Hypertrophy (Rife)... (Rife), Cardiac Hypertrophy (Quan), Heart Energizer (Quan), Heart Tonic (Rife)... Tonic Animals (Rife)
...ity	Green Tea Emulator (Quan), Obesity (Quan), Obesity Overweight (Rife), Fat O... 2 (Rife), Hypothyroidism (Quan), Hypothyroid 2 (Rife)
...ointestinal Problems	Digestive System Support (Quan), Gastroenteritis (Rife), Gastrointestinal Dis... (Rife), Small Intestine (Quan), Intestinal Diseases, (Rife), Intestinal Inflamma... (Rife)

Appendix E: QiCoil Protocols for Canine Extended Home Use

	Each cancer patient and their cancer is slightly different. After the diagnostics have been completed, each owner should contact their health care professional and determine the exact protocol.
	Cancer Program Day #1 (Rife), Cancer Program Day #2 (Rife), Cancer Program Day #3 (Rife), Get Well Soon and Feel Better (Quan)
s	Worms (Quan), Worms, Round (Quan), Worms (Rife), Parasites - Roundworms, General (Rife), Parasites – Tapeworms (Rife), Hookworm Infections (Rife), Whipworm Infections (Rife), Eggs of Worms (Rife)
rms	Parasites – Heartworms (Rife), Dirofilaria Immitis Dog Heartworm (Rife), Parasites Dirofilaria Immitis Dog Heartworm (Rife), Immune Boost Max (Quan)
	Fleas (Rife)
ssues	Kidney Tonic (Quan), Kidneys (Quan), Kidney Function (to Balance and normalize) (Rife), Kidney Insufficiency (Rife), Kidney Infection (Rife), Kidney Function Balance (Rife), Kidney Stimulation (Rife)
ues	Liver Tonic (Quan), Liver (Quan), Liver Support (Rife), Liver Enlargement (Rife), Liver (Rife), Detox Liver Kidneys Lymph Intestines (Rife)
Reaction	10,000, After Jab Detox (Quan), After Jab Detox 2 (Quan), Immune Boost Max (Quan)
y from Surgery	4698, 100, 174, 5000, Pain (Rife), Bruises (Rife), Get Well Soon and Feel Better (Quan), Surgical Pain/Post Op
Dog temp is greater than 102.5)	727, 787, 880, Immune Boost Max (Quan), Get Well Soon and Feel Better (Quan)
d Dog	Locomotor Ataxia, Muscle Failure (Rife), Paralysis (Rife), Ataxia of Muscles (Rife), Inflammation (Rife), Support Joint Health (Quan), Lumbar Vertebra (Rife), Backache (Rife), Numbness, Arms, Fingers (Rife), Nerves, Inflammation (Rife)

Appendix E: QiCoil Protocols for Canine Extended Home Use

ary Tract Infections 727.5, 802, Immune Boost Max (Quan), 146, 4698

Appendix F: QiCoil Frequencies Feline

Treatments (Animal Health Care Professional In House Treatments)

Arthritis	Support Joint Health (Quan), 4698, 570, 146, 1468
Diarrhea	Digestive System Support (Quan), 727.5, 787, 880, 440
Lameness	Support Joint Health (Quan), 1468, 2336, 130, 787
Lack of Appetite	Regenerate (Quan), Cell Metabolism Regenerator (Quan), Get Well So[on], Feel Better (Quan)
Ear Infection	727.5, Colloidal Silver Emulator (Quan), Immune Boost (Quan), 802, 8[...]
Itchy Skin	Psoriasis (Rife), Pruritus (Rife), Dandruff (Rife), Erysipelas (Rife), Immu[ne] Boost Max (Quan)
Mouth Issues	Dental Infections and Cavitations (Rife), Periodontal Disease (Rife), G[um] inflammation (Rife), Tooth Decay (Rife)
Urinary Tract Infections	727.5, 802, Immune Boost Max (Quan), 146, 4698
Diabetes	diabetes (Rife), Detox (Quan), Inflammation (Quan), Pancreatic Disea[se] (Quan), Pancreas (Quan)
Kidney Disease	Kindey Tonic (Quan), Kidneys (Quan), Kidney Tonic (Quan), Nephritis, Inflammation (Quan)
Obesity	70, 460, 459.12, 425.88, Detox (Quan), Distended Stomach (Quan)

Appendix G: QiCoil Frequencies Equine

Treatments (Animal Health Care Professional In House Treatments)

Condition	Frequencies
Arthritis	Support Joint Health (Quan), 4698, 570, 146, 1468
Diarrhea	Digestive System Support (Quan), 727.5, 787, 880, 440
Lameness	Support Joint Health (Quan), 1468, 2336, 130, 787
Itchy Skin	Psoriasis (Rife), Pruritus (Rife), Dandruff (Rife), Erysipelas (Rife), Immune Boost (Quan)
Laminitis	Regenerate (Quan), Cell Metabolism Regenerator (Quan), Get Well Soon & Feel Better (Quan), Lymphatic System (Rife), Toxin Elimination (Rife)
Sore Back	Disk, Slipped (Quan), Injuries (Quan), Trauma, Injury, Shock (Quqn), Arthr (Quan), Osteoarthritis (Quan)
Colic	Get Well Soon and Feel Better (Quan), Dyspepsia (Quan) Stomach, Cramp (Quan), Small Intestine (Quan), Intestines, Spasms (Quan)
COPD	Immune Boost (Quan), Allergies (Quan), Detox (Quan), Toxin Elimination (Quan), Asthma (Rife), Breathing Problems (Rife), Lungs (Rife),
Ulcers	Anxiety (Quan), Acidosis (Rife), Digestive System Support (Quan), Stomach Disorders (Rife), Distended Stomach (Rife), Hyperacidity Stomach 1 (Rife
Parasites	Worms (Quan),
PM	Immune Boost (Quan), Qi Energy Flow-Liver Cleanse (Quan), Nerves, Inflammation (Rife), Nervous System Tonic (Rife)

Appendix H: QiCoil Long Equine Therapies

Arthritis	Support Joint Health (Quan),4698, 570, 146, 1468
Diarrhea	Digestive System Support (Quan), 727.5,787,880,440
Lameness	Support Joint Health (Quan), 1468, 2336, 130, 787
Itchy Skin	Psoriasis (Rife), Pruritus (Rife), Dandruff (Rife), Erysipelas (Rife),Boost (Quan)
Laminitis	Regenerate (Quan), Cell Metabolism Regenerator (Quan), Get Well Soon and Feel Better (Quan), Lymphatic System (Rife), Toxin Elimination (Rife)
Sore Back	Disk, Slipped (Quan), Injuries (Quan), Trauma, Injury, Shock (Quqn), Arthritis (Quan), Osteoarthritis (Quan), Backache (Quan), Lumbar Vertebra (Quan), Rickets, Vitamin D and Snlight (Quan), Spondylitis (Quan), Inflammation (Quan)
Colic	Get Well Soon and Feel Better (Quan), Dyspepsia (Quan)Stomach, Cramps (Quan), Small Intestine (Quan), Intestines, Spasms (Quan), Abdominal Cramps (Quan)Digestion (Quan), Cramps , Abdominal (Quan)Constipation (Quan), Abdominal Pain (Quan), Colic (Stomach and Colon Pain)(Quan)
COPD	Immune Boost (Quan), Allergies (Quan), Detox (Quan), Toxin Elimination (Quan), Asthma (Rife), Breathing Problems (Rife), Lungs (Rife),
Ulcers	Lymphatic System- Circulation and Drainage (Quan), Digestive System Support (Quan), Qi Energy Boost (Quan), Relieve Anxiety (Quan), Anxiety (Quan), Acidosis (Rife), Stomach Disorders (Rife), Distended Stomach (Rife), Hyperacidity Stomach 1 (Rife)
Parasites	Worms (Quan),
EPM	Immune Boost (Quan), Qi Energy Flow-Liver Cleanse (Quan), Nerves, Inflammation (Rife), Nervous System Tonic (Rife)
EOTRH (dental issues)	

Appendix I: Frequencies for some common animal issues

A

Abdominal inflammation   Dogs, Horses, Cats, Other Animals
1. 1.25 Hz
2. 880 Hz   Acute – 465, 440, 125, 1.25
3. 1800 Hz
4. 2489 Hz   Chronic – 2720, 2170, 1600, 1550

Determine the underlying factors and treat for that condition as well

Abrasions   Dogs, Horses, Cats, Other Animals
1. 363 Hz
2. 9 Hz   Acute – 727, 465, 200, 20
3. 73 Hz
4. 42 Hz   Chronic – 10000, 880, 787, 727

Abscess   Dogs, Horses, Cats, Other Animals
1. 42 Hz
2. 190 Hz   Acute-880, 500, 190, 20
3. 444 Hz
4. 1865 Hz   Chronic-10000, 5000, 2720, 2170

Acne   Cats
1. 20 Hz
2. 83 Hz   Acute-564, 450, 444, 428
3. 363 Hz
4. 426 Hz   Chronic-5000, 1800, 1550, 802

Acute Injury   Dogs, Horses, Cats, Other Animals
1. 3 Hz   5) 300 Hz   9) 9 Hz
2. 25 Hz   6) 192 Hz   10) 16 Hz
3. 42 Hz   7) 96 Hz   11) 42 Hz
4. 125 Hz   8) 95 Hz   12) 53 Hz

Addison's disease   Dogs, Horses
1. 21 Hz
2. 59 Hz
3. 666 Hz
4. 2720 Hz

Adhesions (Adhesive Capsulitis)   Horses
1. 8 Hz
2. 42 Hz   Acute- 727, 465, 20, 18
3. 45 Hz
4. 750 Hz   Chronic-10000, 1550, 880, 802

Determine the underlying factors and treat for that condition as well

Adrenal Support   Dogs, Horses, Cats, Other Animals
1. 9 Hz
2. 21 Hz   Acute-465, 95, 20, 10
3. 33 Hz
4. 59 Hz   Chronic-2720, 2128, 1600, 1500

Aflatoxin exposure   Horses

1. 568 Hz
2. 476 Hz   Acute, 344
3. 474 Hz
4. 510 Hz   Chronic-2489, 943

Allergies   Dogs, Horses, Cats, Other Animals
1. 16 Hz
2. 21 Hz   Acute-775, 727, 330, 3
3. 53 Hz
4. 73 Hz   Chronic-10000, 843, 787, 465

Alopecia   Dogs, Horses, Cats, Other Animals
1. 9 Hz
2. 25 Hz   Acute-727, 465, 146, 20
3. 100 Hz
4. 727 Hz   Chronic-1552, 880, 800, 787

Alpha Waves   Dogs, Horses, Cats, Other Animals
1. 8 Hz
2. 14 Hz
3. 8 Hz
4. 14 Hz

The neurons in the parietal lobes produce the biochemical acetylcholine and its associated alpha waves, which control brain speed and relative brain age.

Anal Glands   Dogs
    1. 20 Hz
    2. 72 Hz   Acute-35, 15, 14, 9.5
    3. 95 Hz
    4. 465 Hz   Chronic-1865, 826, 773, 685

Anemia   Dogs, Horses, Cats, Other Animals
    1. 26 Hz
    2. 73 Hz
    3. 45 Hz
    4. 33 Hz
    5. 1084 Hz
    6. 5829 Hz

Anhydrosis   Horses
    1. 465 Hz   7. 787 Hz
    2. 880 Hz   8. 1800 Hz
    3 428 Hz   9. 464 Hz
    4 664 Hz   10. 727 Hz
    5 1550 Hz   11 2720 Hz
    6 3554 Hz   12. 5000 Hz

Anosmia (loss of smell)   Dogs
    1. 10000
    2. 800
    3. 465
    4. 20

Anthrax   Other Animals
    1. 1354
    2. 768   Acute-633, 500, 465, 414
    3. 465
    4. 414   Chronic-1370, 1365, 768, 633

Antiviral   Dogs, Horses, Cats, Other Animals
    1. 768
    2. 660   Acute-786, 768, 523, 333
    3. 523
    4. 333   Chronic-2489, 788, 786, 465

Aortic Emboli   Cats, Horses
    1. 9.39 Hz
    2. 33 Hz
    3. 40 Hz
    4. 465 Hz

Arrhythmias — Dogs
1. 9 Hz
2. 33 Hz
3. 59 Hz
4. 6937 Hz

Arthritis — Dogs, Horses, Cats, Other Animals
1. 16 Hz
2. 880 Hz — Acute-40, 28, 15, 2.5
3. 6568 Hz
4. 7683 Hz — Chronic-10000, 5000, 1664, 880
5. 9 Hz
6. 42 Hz
7. 53 Hz

Asthma — Dogs, Horses, Cats, Other Animals
1. 16 Hz
2. 21 Hz — Acute-522, 500, 444, 440
3. 2170 Hz
4. 6458 Hz — Chronic-2720, 2000, 1865, 1283

Atrophy — Dogs, Horses, Cats, Other Animals
1. 9 Hz
2. 16 Hz
3. 42 Hz
4. 53 Hz

Ataxia — Dogs, Horses, Cats, Other Animals
1. 2170
2. 1600 — Acute-125, 95 72, 20
3. 880
4. 444 — Chronic-272, 2170, 1800, 1500

Autoimmune Disorder — Dogs, Horses, Cats, Other Animals
1. 1550
2. 880 — Acute-250, 146, 28, 9.5
3. 727
4. 650 — Chronic-10000, 1850, 1550, 1500

B

Back Pain   Dogs, Horses, Cats, Other Animals
1. 9 Hz.
2. 16 Hz   Acute-465, 305, 212, 33
3. 42 Hz
4. 3 Hz   Chronic-10000, 1550, 802, 787

Beta Waves   Dogs, Horses, Cats, Other Animals
1. 14 Hz
2. 50 Hz
3. 14 Hz
4. 50 Hz

Every part of the body is connected through nerve cells that lead to the frontal lobes. These connections allow the body to receive sensation of heat, cold and touch. The frontal lobes control movement and response to stimuli, as well as help to shape personality. Beta brain waves are created in the frontal lobes from neurons that produce the biochemical dopamine.

Bites (Insect and/or animal)   Dogs, Horses, Cats, Other Animals
1. 2709 Hz
2. 3239 Hz   Acute- 724
3. 4139 Hz
4. 5612 Hz   Chronic- 880, 787, 690
5. 376 Hz
6. 465 Hz
7. 727 Hz
8. 5000 Hz

Bloating   Dogs
1. 55 Hz
2. 324 Hz
3. 880 Hz
4. 2366 Hz
5. 6921 Hz
6. 70655 Hz

Blood Pressure (High)   Dogs, Horses, Cats, Other Animals
1. 9.19 Hz
2. 33 Hz   Acute – 95, 20, 9.25, 6
3. 728 Hz
4. 10,000 Hz   Chronic – 10000, 880, 787, 727

Blood Pressure (Low)　　　　　　　　　　　　Dogs, Horses, Cats, Other Animals
1. 9.19 Hz
2. 33 Hz　　　　　　　　　　Acute – 522, 330, 148, 20
3. 728 Hz
4. 10,000 Hz　　　　　　　　Chronic – 10000, 999, 727, 555

Blood Sugar Balance　　　　　　　　　　　　Dogs, Horses, Cats, Other Animals
1. 9.39 Hz
2. 20 Hz　　　　　　　　　　Acute – 648, 624, 464, 440
3. 53 Hz
4. 733 Hz　　　　　　　　　　Chronic – 10000, 1552, 880, 600

Bone　　　　　　　　　　　　　　　　　　　Dogs, Horses, Cats, Other Animals
1. 20 Hz
2. 45 Hz
3. 3594 Hz
4. 8687 Hz

Bowed Tendons　　　　　　　　　　　　　　Horses
1. 1.2 Hz
2. 20.5 Hz　　　　　　　　　Acute – 72, 28, 26, 1.5
3. 250 Hz
4. 2720 Hz　　　　　　　　　Chronic – 880, 802, 786, 452

Bradycardia　　　　　　　　　　　　　　　Dogs, Horses, Cats, Other Animals
1. 4 Hz
2. 9 Hz
3. 33 Hz
4. 60 Hz

Bronchitis　　　　　　　　　　　　　　　　Dogs, Horses, Cats, Other Animals
1. 21 Hz
2. 83 Hz　　　　　　　　　　Acute-727, 72, 20, 9.5
3. 801 Hz
4. 6458 Hz　　　　　　　　　Chronic-7344, 3672, 1234, 880

Bruises　　　　　　　　　　　　　　　　　Dogs, Horses, Cats, Other Animals
1. 25 Hz
2. 42 Hz　　　　　　　　　　Acute-465, 110, 9.5, 9
3. 363 Hz
4. 8687 Hz　　　　　　　　　Chronic-10000, 880, 787, 727

Bucked shins
1. 45 Hz
2. 20 Hz
3 9 Hz
4 42 Hz

Burns
1. 8 Hz
2. 12 Hz
3. 28 Hz
4. 45 Hz
5. 2647 Hz

Bursitis
1. 9 Hz
2. 16 Hz
3. 1442 Hz
4. 6568 Hz
5. 42 Hz
6. 53 Hz

Horses
5. 3594 Hz
6. 687 Hz
7. 16 Hz
8. 53 Hz

Dogs, Horses, Cats, Other Animals

Acute – 465, 200, 190, 26

Chronic-10000, 880, 787, 465

Dogs, Horses, Cats, Other Animals

Acute-60, 40, 26, 15

Chronic-2000, 1664, 1550, 810.25

C

Calcium Deposits or Formations   Dogs, Horses, Cats, Other Animals
1. 5 Hz
2. 20 Hz
3. 250 Hz
4. 43 Hz
5. 20 Hz
6. 465 Hz
7. 1.25 Hz

Candida   Dogs, Horses, Cats, Other Animals
1. 21 Hz
2. 762 Hz   Acute-675, 450, 414, 25
3. 880 Hz
4. 1146 Hz   Chronic-1403, 1146, 709, 675

Cancer   Dogs, Horses, Cats, Other Animals
1. 2180 Hz
2. 2008 Hz   Acute-465, 433, 418, 120
3. 2001 Hz
4. 1050 Hz   Chronic-6064, 3524, 3176, 2135

Place the preprogrammed head over the brain or spinal cord related to the affected area and the programmed head over the affected area of the body for (60-420 seconds).

Canine Cognitive Dysfunction   Dogs
1. 7.69 Hz   7. 33 Hz
2. 37 Hz   8. 9 Hz
3. 8 Hz   9. 13 Hz.
4. 15 Hz   10. 60 Hz
5. 61 Hz   11. 993 Hz
6. 30 Hz   12. 34 Hz

Canine Distemper   Dogs
1. 20 Hz
2. 73 Hz   Acute-1862, 465, 432, 8
3. 465 Hz
4. 728 Hz   Chronic-5611 4014, 3448, 2180
5. 20 Hz
6. 125 Hz
7. 10,000 Hz
8. 13011 Hz

Canine Kerititis Sicca   Dogss
    1. 436 Hz
    2. 595 Hz
    3. 775 Hz
    4. 952 Hz

Canine Parvovirus   Dogs
    1. 20 Hz
    2. 73 Hz   Acute-2008, 465, 432, 8
    3. 465 Hz
    4. 728 Hz   Chronic-5611, 3448, 3347, 2929
    5. 16 Hz
    6. 66 Hz
    7. 83 Hz
    8. 2949 Hz

Capped elbow / Shoe Boil / Hygroma of the Elbow   Horses
    1. 9 Hz
    2. 16 Hz   Acute-465, 110, 9.5
    3. 1,442 Hz
    4. 6,568 Hz   Chronic-10000, 880, 787, 727
    5. 42 Hz
    6. 53 Hz

Capped Hock   Horses
    1. 9 Hz
    2. 16 Hz   Acute-465, 110, 9.5, 9
    3. 1,442 Hz
    4. 6,568 Hz   Chronic-10000, 880, 787, 727
    5. 42 Hz
    6. 53 Hz

Capsulitis   Dogs, Horses, Cats, Other Animals
    1. 8 Hz
    2. 42 Hz   Acute-787, 776, 727, 465
    3. 45 Hz
    4. 750 Hz   Chronic-10000, 5000, 880, 802

Cartilage   Dogs, Horses, Cats, Other Animals
    1. 20 Hz
    2. 690 Hz
    3. 787 Hz
    4. 2720 Hz

Cat Scratch Fever   Cats
    1. 967Hz
    2. 786Hz   Acute-654, 465, 364, 379
    3. 645Hz
    4. 379Hz   Chronic-6878, 967, 845, 840

Cataracts   Dogs, Horses, Cats, Other Animals
    1. 81 Hz
    2. 660 Hz   Acute-333, 148, 20, 6.25
    3. 784 Hz
    4. 6147 Hz Causticum   Chronic-2010, 1335, 999, 774

Check Ligament Sprain/Muscle-Tendon Strain   Horses
    1. 4.9 Hz
    2. 9.19 Hz   Acute-465, 26, 20, 1.5
    3. 125 Hz
    4. 2720 Hz   Chronic-2720, 465, 125, 16

Chronic Fatigue   Dogs, Horses, Cats, Other Animals
    1. 21 Hz
    2. 33 Hz   Acute-410, 230, 14, 9.5
    3. 4923 Hz
    4. 6928 Hz   Chronic-2128, 2000, 1850, 589

Circulation (Stimulate Blood Flow)   Dogs, Horses, Cats, Other Animals
    1. 9.39 Hz
    2. 33 Hz   Acute-650, 444, 230, 40
    3. 40 Hz
    4. 465 Hz   Chronic-2720, 2145, 1000, 810.25

Circulation (Balance and Support)   Dogs, Horses, Cats, Other Animals
    1. 15 Hz   Acute-125, 95, 72, 35
    2. 33 Hz
   3. 337 Hz   Chronic- 2000, 1865, 589, 9.5
   4. 6937 Hz

Cirrhosis   Dogs, Horses, Cats, Other Animals
    1. 53 Hz
    2. 465 Hz   Acute-677, 514, 465, 381
    3. 514 Hz
    4. 7952 Hz   Chronic-1550, 1351, 922, 477

Colic   Horses
    1. 20Hz
    2. 72Hz   Acute-776, 465, 440, 20
    3. 727Hz
    4. 880Hz   Chronic-1550, 1500, 880, 832

Colitis   Dogs, Horses, Cats, Other Animals
1. 20 Hz
2. 96 Hz   Acute-787, 465, 440, 20
3. 2,796 Hz
4. 3,791 Hz   Chronic-10000, 1550, 832, 776
5. 97,176 Hz Glutamine

Colitis disease is a long term degenerative condition of the colon. Check for bacteria, virus, fungus, yeast, mold, allergies etc. and eliminate as many offending agents and treat accordingly. You may need to perform brain balance. REMEMBER the colon is the second brain of the body!!!!!!!!!!! Glutamine is an amino acid necessary for rebuilding the colon.

Concussion   Dogs, Horses, Cats, Other Animals
1. 33 Hz   Acute – 37, 33, 13, 8
2. 60 Hz
3. 8687 Hz Arnica Montana   Chronic – 993, 61, 60, 15
4. 6243 Hz Natrum Muriaticum

Congestion   Dogs, Horses, Cats, Other Animals
1. 20 Hz
2. 125 Hz
3. 10,000 Hz
4. 13011 Hz
5. 7048 Hz

Congestive Heart Failure (CHF)   Dogs
1. 9.19 Hz
2. 33 Hz   Acute-80, 33, 20, 8
3. 2,296 Hz Arginine
4. 6,937 Hz Crataegus Oxycantha   Chronic-3000, 880, 160, 95

Conjunctivitis   Dogs, Horses, Cats, Other Animals
1. 432 Hz
2. 722 Hz   Acute-72, 48, 26, 1.5
3. 822 Hz
4. 1,246 Hz   Chronic-5500, 683, 452, 304
5. 5,457 Hz

Constipation   Dogs, Horses, Cats, Other Animals
1. 53 Hz
2. 87 Hz   Acute-727, 465, 422, 20
3. 3,402 Hz
4. 22,961 Hz   Chronic-1550, 880, 787, 776

Coronitis — Horses
1. 9 Hz
2. 16 Hz — Acute-333, 304, 26, 1.5
3. 42 Hz
4. 2720 Hz — Chronic-10000, 5500, 1550, 683

Cramps, Muscle — Dogs, Horses, Cats, Other Animals
1. 6.8 Hz
2. 125 Hz — Acute-190, 95, 72, 20
3. 600 Hz
4. 760 Hz — Chronic-10000, 5000, 776, 465

Crepitus — Dogs, Horses, Cats, Other Animals
1. 8 Hz
2. 42 Hz — Acute-40, 25, 15, 10
3. 45 Hz
4. 750 Hz — Chronic- 2000, 1664, 999, 810.25
5. 9 Hz
6. 16 Hz
7. 42 Hz
8. 53 Hz

Cunean Tendonitis / Bursitis — Horse
1. 9 Hz
2. 16 Hz — Acute-28, 15, 10, 3
3. 1,442 Hz
4. 6,568 Hz — Chronic-10000, 1550 880, 7.75
5. 42 Hz
6. 53 Hz

Curb (Plantar Ligament Sprain) — Horse
1. 4.9 Hz
2. 9.19 Hz — Acute-465, 26, 20, 1.5 up to 20 minutes
3. 125 Hz
4. 2720 Hz

Cuts — Dogs, Horses, Cats, Other Animals
1. 3 Hz
2. 16 Hz — Acute- 727, 465, 26, 20
3. 24 Hz
4. 111 Hz — Chronic – 5000, 2720, 887, 880

Cushing's Syndrome — Dogs, Horses, Cats
1. 9 Hz
2. 21 Hz
3. 33Hz
4. 59 Hz

D

Decubital Ulcers   Dogs, Horses, Cats, Other Animals
    1. 42 Hz
    2. 190 Hz   Acute-465, 95, 72, 20
    3. 444 Hz
    4. 1,865 Hz   Chronic-10000, 2950, 1000, 832

Delta Waves   Dogs, Horses, Cats, Other Animals
    1. 3 Hz
    2. 4 Hz
    3. 3 Hz
    4. 4 Hz

The occipital lobes regulate the brain's ability to rest and resynchronize by producing the biochemical serotonin and its resulting delta waves. Serotonin provides a healing, nourishing, satisfied feeling to the brain and body.

Dermatomal Dermatitis   Dogs
    1. 6.3 Hz
    2. 9.19 Hz   Acute-333, 304, 125, 72
    3. 1550 Hz
    4. 2127 Hz   Chronic-5500, 3176, 1000, 1865
    5. 7,556 Hz
    6. 6,361 Hz
    7. 9,866 Hz

Detoxification   Dogs, Horses, Cats, Other Animals
    1. 1550 Hz
    2. 832 Hz   Acute-465, 125, 72, 6.25
    3. 760 Hz
    4. 625 Hz   Chronic-2128, 880, 787, 685

Diabetes   Dogs, Horses, Cats, Other Animals
    1. 9.39 Hz   Acute – 484, 465, 35, 6.75
    2. 20 Hz
    3. 53 Hz   Chronic – 4000, 2128, 2013, 1850
    4. 733 Hz

Diabetic Neuropathy 1   Dogs, Horses, Cats, Other Animals
- 1, 9 Hz
- 2. 16 Hz   Acute – 125, 95, 72, 10
- 3, 42 Hz
- 4. 53 Hz   Chronic – 5000, 1050, 832, 78
- 5. 3.9 Hz
- 6. 728 Hz
- 7. 833 Hz
- 8. 2720 Hz

Diarrhea   Dogs, Horses, Cats, Other Animals
- 1. 16 Hz   Acute – 776, 727, 465, 20
- 2. 66 Hz
- 3. 83 Hz   Chronic – 5000, 1550, 786, 690
- 4. 2949 Hz

Diskospondylitis   Dogs, Horses, Cats, Other Animals
- 1. 5 Hz
- 2. 20 Hz   Acute – 28, 26, 20, 1.5
- 3. 43 Hz
- 4. 465 Hz   Chronic – 1000, 1550, 683, 452
- 5. 9 Hz
- 6. 16 Hz
- 7. 42 Hz
- 8. 2720 Hz

Diskopondylitis(Ankalosing)   Dog
- 1. 3000
- 2. 1550   Acute-95, 60, 35, 14
- 3. 727
- 4. 428   Chronic-3040, 2000, 1550, 810.25

Disk-Herniated   Dog, Cat
- 1. 10000
- 2. 2720
- 3. 787
- 4. 465

E

Echinococcinum (tapeworms) — Dogs, Horses, Cats, Other Animals
1. 623Hz
2. 542Hz
3. 465Hz
4. 164Hz

Eczema — Dogs, Horses, Cats, Other Animals
1. 5000Hz
2. 999Hz   Acute-465, 120, 20, 15
3. 707Hz
4. 664Hz   Chronic-10000, 5000, 2720, 2128

Electrolyte Levels (to improve) — Dogs, Horses, Cats, Other Animals
1. 10000Hz
2. 465Hz
3. 20Hz
4. 8Hz

Edema — Dogs, Horses, Cats, Other Animals
1. 21 Hz
2. 33 Hz   Acute – 444, 440, 148, 6.25
3. 43 Hz
4. 5000 Hz   Chronic – 10000, 5000, 787, 880

Emphysema — Dogs, Horses, Cats, Other Animals
1. 20 Hz
2. 660 Hz   Acute – 465, 120, 80, 20
3. 690 Hz
4. 727 Hz   Chronic – 7344, 3672, 1234, 787

Endometriosis — Dogs, Horses, Cats, Other Animals
1. 10 Hz
2. 537 Hz   Acute – 620, 514, 465, 461
3. 802 Hz
4. 1552 Hz   Chronic – 922, 788, 765, 625

Epicondylitis — Dogs, Horses, Cats, Other Animals
1. 1550
2. 880   Acute-250, 160, 26, 1.5
3. 802
4. 787   Chronic-10000, 3040, 1550, 727

Exertional myositis *(Tying Up, Exertional rhabdomyelitis, Monday morning sickness, Azoturia)*

Horses

1. 9 Hz
2. 16 Hz   Acute – 48, 26, 20, 1.5
3. 42 Hz
4. 53 Hz   Chronic – 10000, 1550, 832, 776

Erysipelas   Other Animals

1. 5000
2. 1550   Acute – 660, 616, 465, 20
3. 727
4. 845   Chronic – 10000, 2000, 1550, 880

F

Facet syndrome   Dogs, Horses, Cats, Other Animals
1. 9 Hz.
2. 16 Hz   Acute – 48, 26, 20, 1.5
3. 42 Hz
4. 3 Hz   Chronic – 10000, 1550, 832, 776

Facial Paralysis   Dogs, Horses, Cats, Other Animals
1. 16 Hz   6. 61 Hz
2. 200 Hz   7. 60 Hz
3. 37 Hz   8. 33 Hz
4. 2557 Hz   9. 15 Hz
5. 2709 Hz   10. 13 Hz

FeLV / FIV   Cats
1. 22 Hz
2. 144 Hz
3. 249 Hz
4. 428 Hz

Fibrocartilagenous emboli   Dogs
1. 9.39 Hz
2. 33 Hz   Acute – 125, 95, 72, 48
3. 40 Hz
4. 465 Hz   Chronic – 10000, 802, 683, 452

Fibrotic myopathy   Horses
1. 8 Hz
2. 16 Hz   Acute – 465, 428, 146, 18
3. 45 Hz
4. 363 Hz   Chronic – 999, 555, 522, 465
5. 9 Hz
6. 42 Hz
7. 53 Hz

Fistula   Dogs Horses
1. 2170
2. 1800   Acute-802, 787, 776, 550
3. 878
4. 844   Chronic-2489, 2128, 1600, 1122

FIV   Cats
   1. 73 Hz
   2. 238 Hz
   3. 683 Hz
   4. 2420 Hz

Food Intolerance   Dogs, Cats, Horses
   1. 16 Hz
   2. 21 Hz
   3. 53 Hz
   4. 73 Hz
   5. 16 Hz
   7. 66 Hz
   8. 83 Hz
   9. 2949 Hz

Founder– Thyroid (Hypo)   Horses
   1. 160 Hz
   2. 531 Hz   Acute - 48, 26, 20, 1.5
   3. 756 Hz
   4. 5311 Hz   Chronic – 10000, 1550, 832, 776

Fracture   Dogs, Horses, Cats, Other Animals
   1. 20 Hz
   2. 45 Hz   Acute – 727, 465, 230, 220
   3. 3594 Hz
   4. 8687 Hz   Chronic – 10000, 880, 787, 776

Fungal Infection   Dogs, Horses, Cats, Other Animals
   1. 21 Hz
   2. 762 Hz   Acute – 422, 254, 72, 20
   3. 880 Hz
   4. 1146 Hz   Chronic – 2222, 1550, 1153, 1016

G

Gait Abnormality   Dogs, Horses, Cats, Other Animals
1. 25 Hz
2. 42 Hz
3. 183 Hz
4. 324 Hz

Have the patient walk around the room while playing these frequencies

Gallbladder (general)   Dogs, Cats, Other Animals
1. 55 Hz
2. 743 Hz   Acute – 16, 13, 9, 1
3. 800 Hz
4. 1550 Hz   Chronic – 458, 55, 53, 38

Gallbladder (stones)   Dogs, Cats, Other Animals
1. 20 Hz
2. 55 Hz   Acute – 16, 13, 9, 1
3. 660 Hz
4. 1552 Hz   Chronic – 458, 55, 53, 38

Gangrene   Dogs, Horses, Cats, Other Animals
1. 5000 Hz
2. 787 Hz   Acute-465, 73, 40, 20
3. 465 Hz
4. 73 Hz   Chronic-5000, 2720, 880, 727

Gingivitis   Dogs, Cats
1. 660 Hz
2. 880 Hz   Acute – 522, 465, 444, 20
3. 1865 Hz
4. 2720 Hz   Chronic – 2720, 2489, 2008, 1800

Glaucoma   Dogs, Horses, Cats, Other Animals
1. 660 Hz
2. 787 Hz   Acute - 633, 125, 81, 60
3. 880 Hz
4. 1830 Hz   Chronic – 10000, 784, 496, 440

Gluomerulonephritis - See Kidney

H

Head Pressing (Right Side)　　　　　　　　Dogs, Horses, Cats, Other Animals
1. 4 Hz
2. 9.5 Hz　　　　　　　　Acute – 35, 26, 15, 9.5
3. 160 Hz 120
4. 2366 Hz b　　　　　　Chronic – 999, 555, 410, 333

Head Pressing (Left Side)　　　　　　　　Dogs, Horses, Cats, Other Animals
1. 4 Hz 180
2. 9.5 Hz　　　　　　　　Acute – 35, 26, 15, 9.5
3. 160 Hz
4. 2792 Hz　　　　　　　Chronic – 999, 555, 410, 333

Headache (General)　　　　　　　　Dogs, Horses, Cats, Other Animals
1. 4 Hz
2. 9.5 Hz　　　　　　　　Acute – 35, 26, 15, 9.5
3. 160 Hz
4. 6243 Hz Natrum Muriaticum　　Chronic – 999, 555, 410, 333

Head Injury　　　　　　　　Dogs, Horses, Cats, Other Animals
1. 3000
2. 787　　　　　　　　Acute-522, 465, 72, 5
3. 522
4. 465　　　　　　　　Chronic-10000, 30000, 880, 727

Heart　　　　　　　　60 to 180 Seconds
1. 9 Hz　　　　　　　　Acute – 95, 73, 20, 4
2. 33 Hz
3. 2296 Hz　　　　　　Chronic – 3000, 880, 787, 727
4. 6937 Hz
5. 4 Hz
6. 37 Hz
7. 444 Hz
8. 5385 Hz

Heartworms　　　　　　　　Dogs, Cats
1. 2322Hz
2. 799　　　　　　　　Acute-543, 535, 465, 200
3. 535
4. 200　　　　　　　　Chronic-2322, 1077, 799, 543

Hematoma   Dogs, Horses, Cats, Other Animals
   1. 25 Hz
   2. 42 Hz   Acute – 465, 110, 9.5, 9
   3. 363 Hz
   4. 8687 Hz   Chronic – 10000, 880, 787, 727

Hemorrhoids   Dogs, Horses
   1. 4474
   2. 1550   Acute-802, 774, 727, 465
   3. 880
   4. 447   Chronic-6117, 4474, 802, 774

Hepatitis   Dogs, Horses, Cats, Other Animals
   1. 3,791 Hz
   2. 346 Hz   Acute –317, 28
   3. 414 Hz
   4. 465 Hz   Chronic – 1550, 1351, 992, 802
   5. 578 Hz
   6. 329 Hz
   7. 334 Hz
   8. 477 Hz
   9. 753 Hz
   10. 779 Hz
   11. 224 Hz

Hives   Dogs, Horses, Cats, Other Animals
   1. 6.3 Hz
   2. 95 Hz   Acute – 522, 465, 146, 5
   3. 125 Hz
   4. 148 Hz   Chronic – 1800, 880, 787, 776

Hoof Wall Cracks   Horses
   1. 95 Hz
   2. 2720 Hz
   3. 3040 Hz
   4. 10,000 Hz

Hormone Balance   Dogs, Horses, Cats, Other Animals
    1. 4 Hz
    2. 59 Hz
    3. 73 Hz
    4. 97 Hz
    5. 21 Hz
    6. 53 Hz
    7. 59 Hz
    8. 10 Hz
    9. 141 Hz

Horner's syndrome - See eye and balance the sympathetic and parasympathetic nervous system.

Hyper/Hypo-Thyroid - See Thyroid

Hyper/Hypo-Glycemia – See Pancreas

I

Iliocolitis   Dogs, Horses, Cats, Other Animals
1. 800
2. 727   Acute-96, 64, 25, 9.5
3. 465
4. 20   Chronic-2489, 1864, 1552, 732

Immune Enhancement   Dogs, Horses, Cats, Other Animals
1. 20 Hz
2. 73 Hz   Acute – 1862, 465, 432, 8
3. 465Hz
4. 728 Hz   Chronic – 5611, 3347, 2867, 2855

Immune Stimulation – See Spleen and Thymus Indigestion
Dogs, Horses, Cats, Other Animals
1. 16 Hz
2. 66 Hz   Acute – 125, 95, 72, 5
3. 83 Hz
4. 2949 Hz   Chronic – 10000, 5000, 880, 444

Infection   Dogs, Horses, Cats, Other Animals
1. 20 Hz
2. 73 Hz   Acute – 125, 48, 28, 3.5
3. 625 Hz
4. 787 Hz   Chronic – 5500, 1500, 786, 683

Inflammatory Bowel Disease   Dogs, Horses, Cats, Other Animals
1. 9 Hz
2. 16 Hz   Acute – 48, 26, 20, 1.5
3. 42 Hz
4. 53 Hz   Chronic – 1550, 802, 683, 452
5. 20 Hz
6. 96 Hz
7. 2796 Hz
8. 6939 Hz

Inflammation   Dogs, Horses, Cats, Other Animals
1. 9 Hz
2. 16 Hz   Acute – 48, 26, 20, 1.5
3. 42 Hz
4. 2720 Hz   Chronic – 10000, 1550, 880, 683
5. 53 Hz

Injuries (Acute)   Dogs, Horses, Cats, Other Animals
    1. 25 Hz   Acute – 465, 300, 192, 96
    2. 42 Hz
    3. 125 Hz   Chronic – 10000, 5000, 3040, 3000
    4. 9 Hz
    5. 16 Hz
    6. 53 Hz
    7. 3 Hz

Insect Bites   Dogs, Horses, Cats, Other Animals
    1. 363 Hz   Acute – 727, 724, 465, 376
    2. 690 Hz
    3. 728 Hz   Chronic – 5000, 1550, 880, 724
    4. 9 Hz
    5. 16 Hz
    6. 42 Hz
    7. 53 Hz

Intervertebral Disc Disease   Dogs
    1. 9 Hz.
    2. 16 Hz   Acute-465, 300, 192, 96
    3. 42 Hz
    4. 3 Hz   Chronic-10000, 5000, 3040, 3000

J

Jaundice – See Liver

Joints   Dogs, Horses, Cats, Other Animals
1. 9 Hz
2. 16 Hz   Acute – 48, 26, 20, 1.25
3. 1442 Hz
4. 6568 Hz   Chronic – 880, 786, 683, 452
5. 42 Hz
6. 53 Hz

K

Kidney									Dogs, Horses, Cats, Other Animals
  1. 9.4 Hz
  2. 21 Hz						Acute – 43, 12, 9.25, 1
  3. 523 Hz
  4. 786 Hz						Chronic – 1600, 1550, 1500, 880

Kidney Inflammation (Nephritis, Primary)		Dogs, Horses, Cats, Other Animals
  1. 3000Hz
  2. 880Hz						Acute-73, 40, 20, 10
  3. 688Hz
  4. 490Hz						Chronic-10000, 5000, 1500, 555

Kidney Stones							Dogs
  1. 30.5 Hz
  2. 444 Hz						Acute – 522, 146, 20, 3.5
  3. 690 Hz
  4. 10,000 Hz						Chronic – 6000, 3040, 2489, 999

L

Laminitis   Horses
  1. 15 Hz
  2. 33 Hz   Acute-48, 26, 20, 1.5
  3. 337 Hz
  4. 6937 Hz Crataegus Oxycantha   Chronic-10000, 1550, 766, 465

Large Intestine   Dogs, Horses, Cats, Other Animals
  1. 53 Hz
  2. 87 Hz
  3. 727 Hz   Chronic-10000, 1550, 832, 776
  4. 465 Hz
  5. 751 Hz
  6. 20 Hz
  7. 96 Hz
  8, 440 Hz
  9. 880 Hz

Laryngitis   Dog
  1. 341 Hz
  2. 727 Hz   Acute-72, 48, 26, 20
  3. 880 Hz
  4. 5000 Hz   Chronic-10000, 5500, 1550, 683

Legg-Perthes   Dog
  1. 20 Hz
  2. 45 Hz
  3. 3594 Hz
  4. 8687 Hz
  5. 9.39 Hz
  6. 33 Hz
  7. 40 Hz
  8. 465 Hz

Lick Granulomas Front Limb   Dog, Cat
  1. 9 Hz
  2. 16 Hz   Acute-16, 9, 8, 1
  3. 21 Hz
  4. 36 Hz   Chronic-463, 338, 61, 60

Ligament   Dogs, Horses, Cats, Other Animals
1. 4.9 Hz
2. 9.19 Hz   Acute-192, 190, 96, 95
3. 125 Hz
4. 2720 Hz   Chronic-2720, 465, 300, 192

Liver (Balance and Support)   Dogs, Horses, Cats, Other Animals
1. 53 Hz
2. 537 Hz   Acute-55, 53, 16, 9
3. 55 Hz
4. 751 Hz   Chronic-1552, 802, 727, 465

Low Back Pain   Dogs, Horses, Cats, Other Animals
1. 9 Hz
2. 16 Hz   Acute- 250, 28, 20, 9.5
3. 42 Hz
4. 53 Hz
5. 26 Hz   Chronic- 1550, 880, 802
6. 2720 Hz
7. 5000 Hz
8, 10,000 Hz

Lungs   Dogs, Horses, Cats, Other Animals
1. 9.4 Hz
2. 21 Hz
3. 523 Hz
4. 786 Hz

Lyme Disease   Dogs, Horses
1. 306 Hz
2. 312 Hz   Acute-432, 345, 338, 254
3. 525 Hz
4. 534 Hz   Chronic-6870, 4200, 1455, 797

Lymphatic   Dogs, Horses, Cats, Other Animals
1. 15 Hz
2. 42 Hz   Acute-444, 146, 10, 2.5
3. 146 Hz
4. 522 Hz   Chronic-10000, 5000, 3176, 833

M

Mammary Gland   Dogs, Horses, Cats, Other Animals
    1. 6 Hz
    2. 16 Hz
    3. 42 Hz
    4. 57 Hz

Malabsorbtion Syndrome   Dogs, Horses, Cats, Other Animals
    1. 3000Hz
    2. 1552Hz
    3. 787Hz
    4. 465Hz

Mange   Dogs, Horses, Cats, Other Animals
    1. 774
    2. 693
    3. 465
    4. 253

Menengitis   Dogs, Horses, Cats, Other Animals
    1. 1865Hz
    2. 1550Hz
    3. 822Hz
    4. 423Hz

Mental Fatigue   Dogs, Horses, Cats, Other Animals
    1. 8 Hz
    2. 14 Hz
    3. 8 Hz
    4. 14 Hz

Mold/Fungus-General   Dogs, Horses, Cats, Other Animals
    1. 2411Hz
    2. 1823Hz   Acute-414, 344, 321, 132
    3. 942Hz
    4. 132Hz   Chronic-2411, 1823, 942, 866

Motion Sickness   Dog
    1. 4 Hz
    2. 9 Hz
    3. 33 Hz
    4. 60 Hz

Muscle   Dogs, Horses, Cats, Other Animals
    1. 9 Hz
    2. 16 Hz
    3. 42 Hz
    4. 53 Hz

Muscle Relaxation   Dogs, Horses, Cats, Other Animals
    1. 6000Hz
    2. 465Hz   Acute-304, 240
    3. 120Hz
    4. 20Hz   Chronic- 965, 760

Muscle tremors   Dogs, Horses, Cats, Other Animals
    1. 815Hz
    2. 500Hz   Acute-15, 2.5, 1.5, 1
    3. 465Hz
    4. 15Hz   Chronic-2000, 727

Myositis of any muscle due to overexertion.   Dogs, Horses, Cats, Other Animals

    1. 9 Hz
    2. 16 Hz   Acute-129, 125, 122, 120
    3. 42 Hz
    4. 53 Hz   Chrinic-1169, 1124, 762, 465

N

Neuropathy   Dogs, Horses, Cats, Other Animals
1. 9 Hz
2. 16 Hz   Acute-146, 95, 72, 6.25
3. 42 Hz
4. 53 Hz   Chronic-999, 690, 555, 422
5. 3.9 Hz
6. 728 Hz
7. 833 Hz
8. 2720 Hz

Numbness (lack of proprioception)   Dogs, Horses, Cats, Other Animals
1. 5.5 Hz
2. 764 Hz   Acute-16, 9, 8, 1
3. 833 Hz
4. 2720 Hz   Chronic-463, 383, 61, 60

O

Oral Ulcers   Dogs, Cats. Horses. Other Animals
    1. 234 Hz
    2. 677 Hz   Acute-690, 522, 444, 146
    3. 787 Hz
    4. 6243 Hz Natrum Muriaticum   Chronic-2720, 2489, 787, 727

Lysine (4236 Hz) is an amino acid that is very beneficial for the remission of some viral infections.

Osteoporosis   Dogs, Reptiles
    1. 20 Hz
    2. 600 Hz   Acute-465, 380, 250, 1.25
    3. 660 Hz
    4. 1600 Hz   Chronic-10000, 2720, 1550, 787

Osteoarthritis   Dogs, Cats. Horses. Other Animals
    1. 880Hz
    2. 787Hz   Acute-81, 9, 8, 7
    3. 465Hz
    4. 171Hz   Chronic-10000, 880, 787, 20

Otitis Externa   Dogs, Cats. Horses. Other Animals
    1. 125 Hz
    2. 440 Hz   Acute-465, 482, 174, 20
    3. 720 Hz
    4. 786 Hz   Chronic-5311, 1550, 880, 776

May also treat the patient for candida and/or allergies as needed.

P

Pain   Dogs, Cats. Horses. Other Animals
1. 16 Hz
2. 2720 Hz   Acute-13, 10, 9, 2
3. 8687 Hz
4. 10,000 Hz
5. 95 Hz
6. 2720 Hz   Chronic-5000, 698, 465, 333
7. 3040 Hz
8. 10,000 Hz

Pain - Injury Related Pain (Localized)   Dogs, Cats. Horses. Other Animals
1. 1.1 Hz
2. 20.5 Hz   Chronic-5000, 465, 313
3. 40 Hz
4. 10,000 Hz
5. 3 Hz
6. 25 Hz   Acute-465, 380, 160, 26
7. 42 Hz
8. 125 Hz

Pancreatitis   Dogs
1. 66 Hz
2. 465 Hz   Acute-465, 444, 26, 20
3. 625 Hz
4. 880 Hz   Chronic-10000, 2720, 2489, 2128

Parasympathetic Facilitation   Dogs, Cats. Horses. Other Animals
1. 9 Hz
2. 20 Hz
3. 5000 Hz
4. 10,000 Hz

Parasite   Dogs, Cats. Horses. Other Animals 64 Hz
1. 72 Hz   Acute-125, 112, 96, 64
2. 96 Hz
3. 120 Hz   chronic.2489, 1864, 712, 685
4. 644 Hz
5. 660 Hz
6. 728 Hz
7. 1550 Hz
8. 6297 Hz
9. 7787 Hz
10. 8416 Hz

Pemphigus   Dogs
    1. 893Hz
    2. 694Hz
    3. 665Hz
    4. 465Hz

Pericarditis   Dogs, Cats. Horses. Other Animals
    1. 2170Hz
    2. 1550Hz   Acute-125, 95, 72, 20
    3. 802Hz
    4. 465Hz   Chronic-2720, 1600, 787, 625

Periodontal Disease   Dogs, Cats. Horses. Other Animals
    1. 1600Hz
    2. 802Hz   Acute-625, 600, 380, 47.5
    3. 776 Hz
    4. 465 Hz   Chronic-10000, 1800, 787, 650

Pink Eye (Conjunctivitis)   Cattle,
    1. 432 Hz
    2. 722 Hz   Acute-95, 72, 48, 20
    3. 822 Hz
    4. 1246 Hz   Chronic-5000, 1865, 786, 683

Pneumonia – See Lung, Infection

Pododermatitis   Dogs
    1. 20 Hz
    2. 53 Hz   Acute-48, 26, 20, 1.5
    3. 363 Hz
    4. 465 Hz   Chronic-880, 802, 786, 683

Post Operative Scar Revision   Dogs, Cats. Horses. Other Animals
    1. 8 Hz
    2. 16 Hz   Acute-45, 25, 18, 8
    3. 45 Hz
    4. 363 Hz   Chronic-2720, 1550, 465, 279

Proprioception loss (numbness)   Dogs, Cats. Horses. Other Animals
    1. 5.5 Hz
    2. 764 Hz   Acute-16, 9, 8, 1
    3. 833 Hz
    4. 2720 Hz   Chronic-463, 338, 60, 61

Prostate
1. 10 Hz
2. 33 Hz
3. 100 Hz
4. 9 Hz 120

Psoriasis – See Skin, Liver

Punctures – See Cuts

Dogs

Acute-125, 95, 72, 9

Chronic-2127, 2008, 690, 465

Q

Q Fever
    1. 1062
    2. 720
    3. 549
    4. 129

Goats, Sheep, Cattle

Acute-607, 549, 523, 465

Chronic-1357, 943, 726

R

Rash   Dogs, Cats. Horses. Other Animals
1. 363 Hz
2. 55 Hz 180   Acute-48, 26, 20, 1.5
3. 53 Hz 120
4. 73 Hz 120   Chronic-880, 802, 786, 683

Rectal Prolapse   Dogs, Cats. Horses. Other Animals
1. 20 Hz
2. 660 Hz
3. 727 Hz
4. 4474 Hz

Renal Problems – See Kidney

Relaxation   Dogs, Cats. Horses. Other Animals
1. 6000Hz
2. 465Hz
3. 10Hz
4. 7.75Hz

Respiratory Problems – See Lungs, Bronchitis

Rhinitis   Dogs, Cats. Horses. Other Animals
1. 1500Hz
2. 727Hz   Acute-444, 146, 26, 20
3. 522Hz
4. 440Hz   Chronic-2720, 1550, 880, 1600

S

Scar Tissue Dogs, Cats. Horses. Other Animals
1. 8 Hz
2. 16 Hz Acute-45, 25, 18, 8
3. 45 Hz
4. 363 Hz Chronic-1550, 465, 279, 45

Sciatica Dogs, Cats. Horses. Other Animals
1. 9 Hz
2. 16 Hz Acute-465, 20, 10
3. 42 Hz
4. 53 Hz Chronic-10000, 1550, 787, 727
5. 120 Hz
6. 305 Hz
7. 4678 Hz
8. 5657 Hz

Sebaceous cysts Dogs, Cats. Horses. Other Animals
1. 42 Hz
2. 363 Hz Acute-557, 523, 478, 465
3. 880 Hz
4. 3499 Hz Chronic-880, 787, 727, 660

Seizures Dogs, Cats. Horses. Other Animals
1. 20 Hz
2. 226 Hz
3. 465 Hz
4. 329 Hz
5. 953 Hz

Sinusitis Dogs, Cats. Horses. Other Animals
1. 20 Hz
2. 60 Hz Acute-146, 120, 72, 20
3. 160 Hz
4. 400 Hz Chronic-1862, 1552, 880, 660

Skin Dogs, Cats. Horses. Other Animals
1. 20 Hz
2. 42 Hz
3. 53 Hz5.
4. 125 Hz Chronic-5000, 1500, 1489, 80
5. 363 Hz
6. 465 Hz
7. 800 Hz

Small Intestine   Dogs, Cats. Horses. Other Animals
    1. 20 Hz
    2. 96 Hz   Acute-800, 727, 465, 53
    3. 223 Hz
    4. 728 Hz   Chronic-3000, 1550, 880, 787

Sore Throat – See Throat

Spleen (Immune Stimulation)   Dogs, Cats. Horses. Other Animals
    1. 27.44 Hz
    2. 73 Hz   Acute-465, 146, 35, 20
    3. 727 Hz
    4. 1800 Hz   Chronic-10000, 2720, 2489, 1600

Sprains – See Muscle

Spurs – See Calcium Deposits or Formations

Staph Infection   Dogs, Cattle
    1. 424 Hz
    2. 453 Hz   Acute-550, 453, 465, 424,
    3. 634 Hz
    4. 2600 Hz   Chronic-1109, 1089, 943, 639

Stings – See Bites

Stomach   60 to 240 Seconds
    1. 16 Hz
    2. 66 Hz   Acute-125, 72, 20, 4
    3. 83 Hz
    4. 2949 Hz   Chronic-10000, 2128, 1552, 832

Stomach Ulcer – See Digestion

Strain – See Muscle, Bursitis, acute trauma

Straining to Urinate   Cats, Dogs
    1. 24 Hz
    2. 43 Hz
    3. 2008 Hz
    4. 7498 Hz

Strep Infections   Dogs, Cats. Horses. Other Animals
    1. 232 Hz
    2. 433 Hz   Acute-334, 134, 128, 114
    3. 465 Hz
    4. 1010 Hz   Chronic-1902, 1415, 1266, 1202

Stye   Dogs, Cats. Horses. Other Animals
    1. 81 Hz
    2. 350 Hz   Acute-727, 465, 453, 20
    3. 660 Hz
    4. 787 Hz   Chronic-880, 787, 727, 465
    5. 2,709 Hz

Sunburns   Pigs
    1. 8 Hz
    2. 12 Hz
    3. 28 Hz
    4. 45 Hz
    5. 2,647 Hz

Surgery pre-op/post-op   Dogs, Cats. Horses. Other Animals
    1. 1800Hz
    2. 880Hz   Acute-330, 250, 160, 26
    3. 727Hz
    4. 589Hz   Chronic-3040, 2170, 1500, 589

Surgical Pain (post-op) recovery   Dogs, Cats. Horses. Other Animals
    1. 3000Hz
    2. 2720Hz
    3. 465Hz
    4. 95Hz

Surgery, post-op anesthesia detox   Dogs, Cats. Horses. Other Animals
    1. 555Hz
    2. 465Hz   Acute-333, 146, 6.25, 2.5
    3. 333Hz
    4. 148Hz   Chronic-999, 555, 522, 465

Sympathetic Calming/Balance   Dogs, Cats. Horses. Other Animals
    1. 2.5 Hz
    2. 7.83Hz
    3. 6000 Hz
    4. 465 Hz
    5. 10 Hz
    6. 7.75 Hz
    7. 764 Hz
    8. 10,000 Hz

T

Tachycardia   Dogs, Cats. Horses. Other Animals
1. 9 Hz
2. 33 Hz Heart   Acute-160, 80, 73, 4
3. 59 Hz Thyroid
4. 6937 Hz Crataegus Oxycantha   Chronic-3000, 880, 727, 125
5. 1.2 Hz

Teeth   Dogs, Cats. Horses. Other Animals
1. 28 Hz
2. 424 Hz   Acute-465, 522, 444, 146
3. 660 Hz
4. 1552 Hz   Chronic-2489, 1556, 625
5. 28 Hz
6. 728 Hz
7. 802 Hz
8. 2,729 Hz

Tendonmyopathy   Dogs, Horses
1. 1.2 Hz
2. 20.5 Hz   Acute-95, 26, 20, 1.5
3. 250 Hz
4. 2720 Hz   Chronic-5000, 465, 300, 192

Theta Waves   Dogs, Cats. Horses. Other Animals
1. 4 Hz
2. 7 Hz
3. 4 Hz
4. 7 Hz

Throat (Sore)   Dogs, Cats. Horses. Other Animals
1. 440 Hz
2. 690 Hz   Acute-48, 26, 20, 1.5
3. 728 Hz
4. 2720 Hz   Chronic-10000, 1550, 786, 452

Thrush   Horses
1. 464 Hz
2. 660 Hz   Acute-465, 414, 72, 60
3. 728 Hz
4. 34999 Hz   Chronic-2167, 1151, 709, 381

Thyroid (Hyper)   Dogs, Cats. Horses. Other Animals
    1. 3 Hz
    2. 20 Hz   Secondary-465, 160, 3, 1.5
    3. 59 Hz
    4. 160 Hz

Thyroid (Hypo)   Dogs, Cats. Horses. Other Animals
    1. 20 Hz
    2. 59 Hz   Secondary-8000, 465, 35, 12
    3. 802 Hz
    4. 3884 Hz

Thymus Stimulation (Immune stimulation)   Dogs, Cats. Horses. Other Animals
    1. 5000Hz
    2. 880Hz
    3. 727Hz
    4. 20Hz

TMJ   Dogs, Cats. Horses. Other Animals
    1. 4 Hz
    2. 9 Hz
    3. 33 Hz
    4. 60 Hz

Trauma (involves mental and physical damage)   Dogs, Cats. Horses. Other Animals
    1. 5000Hz
    2. 3000Hz   Acute-465, 300, 192, 96
    3. 880Hz
    4. 300Hz   Chronic-10000, 3040, 787, 760

U

Ulcer 　　　　　　　　　　　　　　　　　　Horse
1. 1.1 Hz
2. 664 Hz　　　　　　　　　　　　　　　　Acute-465, 125, 72, 20
3. 802 Hz
4. 2949 Hz　　　　　　　　　　　　　　　　Chronic-2950, 1600, 1600, 802

Ulcerative Colitis　　　　　　　　　　　　　Dogs, Cats. Horses. Other Animals
1. 20 Hz
2. 96 Hz　　　　　　　　　　　　　　　　　Acute727, 465, 440, 20
3. 2796 Hz Podophyllum
4. 6939 Hz Mercurius Corrosivus　　　　　Chronic-10000, 1550, 832, 787

Upper Respiratory Viral Infections　　　　　Dogs, Cats. Horses. Other Animals
1. 20 Hz
2. 125 Hz　　　　　　　　　　　　　　　　Secondary-712, 465, 336, 278
3. 10,000 Hz
4. 13,011 Hz

Urine Leakage (During Sleep)　　　　　　　Dog
1. 24 Hz
2. 787 Hz
3. 2,448 Hz
4. 4,139 Hz

Urine Leakage (While Awake)　　　　　　　Dog
1. 43 Hz
2. 465 Hz　　　　　　　　　　　　　　　　Acute-802, 787, 727, 465
3. 660 Hz
4. 802 Hz　　　　　　　　　　　　　　　　Chronic-10000, 2720, 1550, 880

Urinary Tract Infection (UTI)　　　　　　　Dogs, Cats. Horses. Other Animals
1. 24 Hz
2. 43 Hz　　　　　　　　　　　　　　　　　Acute-125, 48, 26, 1.5
3. 2008 Hz
4. 7498 Hz　　　　　　　　　　　　　　　　Chronic-10000, 1550, 786, 452

V

Veins   Dogs, Cats. Horses. Other Animals
1. 1.2 Hz
2. 28 Hz   Acute-465, 200, 160, 73
3. 53 Hz
4. 250 Hz   Chronic-2000, 1850, 813.6, 428

Venereal Warts   Dogs, Cats. Horses. Other Animals
1. 489 Hz
2. 874 Hz   Acute-907, 690, 495, 466
3. 5657 Hz
4. 9258 Hz   Chronic-2128, 1600, 907, 495

Vomiting   Dogs, Cats
1. 4.9 Hz
2. 83 Hz
3. 5000 Hz
4. 10,000 Hz

W

Watery Discharge from eye   Dogs, Cats. Horses. Other Animals
1. 436 Hz
2. 595 Hz
3. 775 Hz
4. 952 Hz
5. 5,556 Hz

Warts   Dogs, Cats. Horses. Other Animals
1. 466 Hz
2. 728 Hz   Acute-907, 690, 495, 466
3. 915 Hz
4. 2128 Hz   Chronic-2128, 1600, 907, 495

Wellness (overall)   Dogs, Cats. Horses. Other Animals
1. 867.25Hz
2. 465Hz
3. 7.75Hz
4. 6.75Hzx

Wounds   Dogs, Cats. Horses. Other Animals
1. 3 Hz
2. 16 Hz   Acute-193, 190, 96, 95
3. 24 Hz
4. 111 Hz   Chronic-2720, 465, 300, 42

Appendix J: Comparative Cost and Setup Guide
Qi Coil vs. Other PEMF Systems

J.1 Purpose and Scope

This appendix offers comparative data on cost, performance, portability, and clinical integration among leading pulsed-electromagnetic-field (PEMF) and frequency-therapy systems used in chiropractic and veterinary practice.
All pricing reflects 2025 U.S. averages for professional-grade units and includes approximate accessories (power supply, cables, applicators).[1]
Actual cost and field output vary by configuration and firmware version.

J.2 Comparative Hardware Summary

System	Design Type	Field Strength (mT @ 6 in)	Primary Frequency Range (Hz)
Qi Coil Max / Pro System	Toroidal coil + smartphone app	0.8 – 3.5	1 – 1000 (selectable)
Bemer Pro Set	Mat + controller unit	0.5 – 1.0	10 – 33 (fixed waveform)
Magna Wave Julian / Maxx	Inductive loop (industrial)	10 – 30	35
Assisi Loop 2.0 Vet	Fixed coil loop	0.05 – 0.1	2 – 3

System	Approx. Cost (USD)	Portability
Qi Coil Max / Pro System	$1,200 – $2,400	Hand-held / battery-powered (< 2 lb)
Bemer Pro Set	$5,000 – $6,000	Medium (roll-up mat)
Magna Wave Julian / Maxx	$18,000 – $25,000	Large cart (> 40 lb)
Assisi Loop 2.0 Vet	$300 – $700	Small, disposable (≤ 0.5 lb)

Table J1: Hardware comparison among major PEMF devices.

J.3 Performance and Operational Considerations

Criterion	Qi Coil System	Bemer Pro Set	Magna Wave Series	Assisi Loop
Adjustable Frequency Control	App-based (1–1000 Hz, custom sets)	Limited (10–33 Hz)	Manual dial (1–60 Hz)	Fixed (2 – 3 Hz)
Waveform Variety	Sine, square, sawtooth digital modulation	Sinusoidal	Proprietary complex pulsed AC	Exponential decay
Noise / Comfort	Silent	Silent	Audible clicks / heat	Silent
Field Coverage	12 – 24 in radius (2 coils expandable)	40 × 60 cm mat	Localized loop to whole-body	10 cm loop area
Maintenance	None (battery recharge)	Occasional mat cleaning	Coil inspection / service annually	None
Warranty	2 years standard	3 years limited	3 years limited	Single-use / 90 days
Training Required	1–2 hr. orientation	Minimal	Professional certification recommended	Minimal

Table J2: operational comparison by criterion.

J.4 Economic and Return-on-Investment Model

Setting	Typical Use Scenario	Sessions per Week	Fee per Session (USD)	Time to Recoup Investment
Mobile Animal Chiropractor (Qi Coil)	Adjunct therapy 3 – 5 animals per day	15 - 25	$40 – $60	≈ 2–3 months
Equine Facility (Magna Wave)	Daily stall sessions	40 – 60	$75 – $100	≈ 5–8 months
Small Animal Clinic (Bemer or Qi Coil)	Adjunct therapy 2–3 per hour	60 – 80	$30 – $45	≈ 3–4 months
Rehabilitation Hospital (Bemer)	Post-surgical care program	100 +	$50 – $65	≈ 6–9 months

Diagram J1: "Return on Resonance" curve. ROI starts at ≈ 70 sessions for Qi Coil, 150 for Bemer, 400 for Magna Wave.

J.5 Setup and Environmental Guidelines

Grounding: Ensure metal tables, stalls, and mats are earth-grounded to reduce electromagnetic reflection.
Distance: Maintain ≥ 12 in separation from pacemakers, ECG leads, or unshielded electronics.
Ambient Field Check: Use a handheld gaussmeter (< 1 mG background preferred).
EM Noise Mitigation: Switch off Wi-Fi routers and fluorescent fixtures during sessions for optimal coherence.
Power Stability: Use voltage-regulated adapters or battery packs to avoid waveform distortion.
Cleaning / Storage: Keep coils dry, wound loosely, and away from ferromagnetic materials.

J.6 Snapshot: Cost & Ease of Use

Assisi Loop (tPEMF)
  Place loop over/around target area; auto 15-min session then shut-off. Owners can continue at home.   Very easy: push-button, no settings. Great for discharge/home programs and stall rest.   Lowest equipment barrier; per-case consumable model. Clear instructions and fixed dosing favored in veterinary rehab.
  Lowest upfront cost / easiest home compliance: Assisi Loop. One-button, fixed 15-min dosing and clear instructions; ideal for discharge kits (OA, wound, post-op) or remote clients. The trade-off is consumable cost per case as loops exhaust after a set number of cycles.
  Work well for discharge & home care (dogs/cats) where simplicity rules. Fixed 15-min cycles; minimal training. Blankets/loops are largely hands-off once placed.

BEMER (Equine Line)
  Drape powered blanket on the horse; leg cuffs for limbs. Pre-set programs.   Easy once fitted; stable-friendly. Requires charging, fit, and tack compatibility.   Built for horses; polished hardware and presets. Higher upfront cost than loops; good for barns that want a turnkey blanket approach.
  Equine barn turnkey blanket option: BEMER Equine Line. Clean fit-and-forget blanket and cuffs, minimal operator time. High upfront; good for barns that want a branded, preset solution with frequent use.
  BEMER horse-specific design; higher cost but smooth workflow. Blankets/loops are largely hands-off once placed.

MagnaWave (high-output PEMF machines)
  Operator moves coils/paddles over regions for set durations. Often practitioner-provided sessions. Moderate (trained tech) to advanced (settings/attachments). Portable cases exist; power and training matter. MagnaWave markets training/certification and many barns expect it; factor staff time. Clinic revenue model via per-session fees; common in equine barns.

Capital intensive but supports billable sessions; many practices emphasize staff training/certification and sell session packages to horse owners. Attachments expand use (hoof boxes, mats). MagnaWave is hands-on requiring active coil placement and session management.

Qi Coil

Small spiral coil(s) near the target area; app selects programs/frequencies. Easy for owners; light/portable. Requires smartphone/console familiarity. Marketed as PEMF/Rife-style frequencies. Lowest clinic entry price beyond Assisi; parameter transparency varies by package.

Ultra-portable, owner-friendly with broad program lists: Qi Coil. Low-to-mid entry cost; app-driven presets and portability suit small animals and house calls. Ensure clients are comfortable with phone/app operation and that expectations are appropriately set. Qi Coil is hands-off during a run but requires app selection. Qi Coil's app flexibility is powerful but can overwhelm some owners. Provide a printed protocol.

J.7 Practical Workflow Checklist

Select appropriate device (loop, blanket, coil, mat).
Define clinical goal (pain, wound healing, performance recovery).
Baseline assessment (pain scores, lameness, wound size).
Apply in consistent session lengths/frequencies (per device protocols).
Reassess at 2–3 weeks, adjust plan.
Document outcomes for evidence building.
Educate owners: adjunctive, not curative; track comfort and function.

J.8 Summary and Interpretation

PEMF and healing frequency therapies occupy a growing niche in veterinary medicine. Their safety profile is strong, their non-invasive nature suits both home care and clinical rehab, and their appeal to owners can be leveraged for compliance. The checklists above serve as a practical reference, empowering doctors to integrate these modalities responsibly. While controlled research remains uneven, clinicians can apply structured outcome measures, track cases, and contribute to the evidence base.

Qi Coil offers the most flexible frequency selection, smallest footprint, and lowest acquisition cost—ideal for mobile or mixed-species chiropractors.
Bemer excels in standardized human wellness programs but has limited field control.
Magna Wave delivers deep-penetration therapeutic fields for large animals or orthopedic use, at high initial cost and lower portability.
Assisi Loop provides economical, disposable solutions for localized veterinary applications.
Selection depends on practice model, species, mobility, and desired field depth.

Combining systems is permissible when frequencies are complementary and grounding integrity is verified.

1. C. Andrew Bassett et al., "Effects of Pulsing Electromagnetic Fields on Bone Repair," Journal of Bone and Joint Surgery 58-A (1976): 993–1003.
2. James L. Oschman, Energy Medicine: The Scientific Basis (Edinburgh: Churchill Livingstone, 2016).
3. David G. Siskind and Janice B. Riegel, "Economic Evaluation of Adjunct Electromagnetic Therapies in Veterinary Rehabilitation," Veterinary Economics 41 (2024): 55–62.

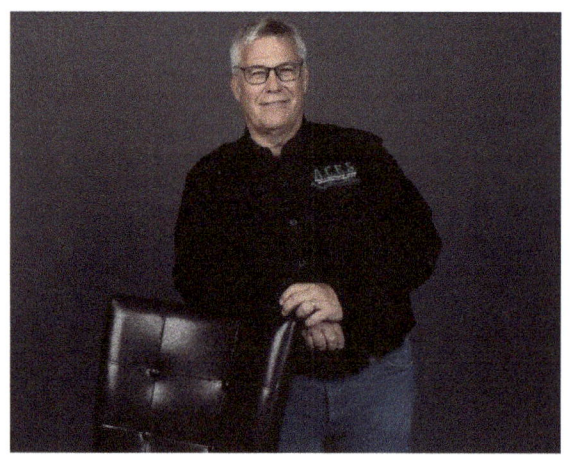

ABOUT THE AUTHOR

Dr. Ormston has spent 30 plus years as a veterinarian and is here to help you determine when your animal's neurological health has been challenged. Removal of these challenges through chiropractic care will help animals overcome their stresses - leading to health, wellness and productivity.

$49.95
ISBN 979-8-9856179-6-2

www.ingramcontent.com/pod-product-compliance
Lightning Source LLC
Chambersburg PA
CBHW042358030426
42337CB00032B/5141